I0092719

In my 20 years as a clinical physical therapist and owner of 39 PT locations, I've evaluated and rehabilitated thousands of bodies—from injured athletes to aging adults just trying to stay mobile. I've seen every fitness trend and gimmick come and go. But what Timothy Ward has created with the Fitness Quadrant is, hands down, the most intelligent, results-driven, and biomechanically sound system I've ever encountered. This program isn't just for one age group—it's for everyone. Whether you're 45 or 75, the way Timothy integrates strength, mobility, cardiovascular conditioning, and recovery is on a level I've never seen. His attention to movement patterns, joint mechanics, and muscle sequencing patterns is masterful. The precision of his biomechanics coaching alone is worth its weight in gold. The Fitness Quadrant is science-based fitness. It's not just effective—it's exceptional.

—Dan Fleury, MPT, Clinical Physical Therapist
20+ Years in Rehabilitation & Human Performance

The changes I have seen in 12 weeks are truly astonishing. No injuries, only 45-minute workouts, I can't understand why someone wouldn't follow this system. The exercise science knowledge I've gained from him is astonishing. And I'm a doctor. It's truly a game changer if you follow it!

—Dr. T, Owner of Dental by Design

First time I have ever had huge success in a fitness routine! At 66 years old I have added 4 lbs. of muscle and lost 13 lbs. of fat in 5 months, and I look dramatically different. A Brilliant system that has now become my lifestyle. If you want to truly battle aging, pay attention. This is a gamechanger.

—Sharry B.

I am a 70-year-old triathlete, racing and training under different programs for 30 years. Tim has been the most effective of them all. For the first time in years, I'm getting faster, sleeping and eating better, lowering my resting heart rate and adding healthy muscle mass. I am also an oral surgeon, seated many hours a day in an ergonomically unfavorable position and Tim's program has protected my posture, core and back.

—Dr. David R., DMD, MS

For 35 years, I battled my weight and fitness. I tried every diet, every workout trend under the sun, every gimmick—and nothing ever stuck. I always ended up back in the same place: frustrated and overweight. Nothing truly made sense… until a friend referred me to Tim. WOW. The way he explains the why behind every move, every protocol, and the bigger payoff completely changed the game for me. For the first time, I wasn't just following a program—I understood it. And that knowledge became the fuel that drove my success. Now, instead of feeling like I'm losing the fight with age, I'm actually aging stronger than I ever thought possible.

—Scott R., Owner
Compass Commercial & Residential Real Estate

Tim's ability to blend advanced strength training, muscle-building strategies, and challenges for balance, flexibility, and endurance makes his system adaptable for anyone—at any age or fitness level. The Fitness Quadrant™ and M.I.T. method are nothing short of remarkable.

—Lauren A.

At 69, Tim has not only transformed my physique and eliminated my shoulder and back problems, but educated me on the science behind the training. His muscle gaining and nutrition coaching has ensured that I optimally fuel my body to support my fitness goals. Tim's dedication to the real science and his clients is evident in his unwavering commitment to their success.

—John S, Retired C-suite Executive

Tim consistently goes above and beyond to tailor programs that are challenging to the individual yet achievable and sustainable. His ability to motivate and inspire is unmatched, creating a positive and supportive environment that fosters personal growth and progress.

—Cindy E.

I'm 56 years old and hate to exercise but realized I need to do something about my health. For years, I repeatedly failed to stick to any workout program. None of them ever really worked. This all changed when I started working with Tim and I'm in better condition than I have been in 20 years.

—Jay H., Property Management Owner

Working as a past U.S diplomat in the Whitehouse and traveling worldwide had me glued to a chair. Tim has been a gamechanger for me with his extensive knowledge and gamechanging systems like the fitness quadrant. He has taught me how to practice fitness properly. I can attest to the fact that this really works! Amazing, unique and super-efficient!

—Betty T., PhD

My personal involvement in coaching and athletics from now Duke basketball players to NBA, I categorize myself as a formidable and knowledgeable athletics guy – until I started training with Tim.

Wow. I cannot emphasize enough the stark difference between his systems and other trainers I have experienced. The goal is always reached. The Fitness Quadrant and M.I.T. training systems are on another level. Gamechanger without a doubt.

—Bill O., Vice President, investments, Stifel

I've been a client of his for 4 years now working twice a week, strength training using his educated study and knowledge of the functions of muscles, bones, and nerves and how they work together to build a strong body.

I was an athlete in my early life and now older, keeping my body healthy and strong is essential to good living. I feel strong and many of the aches and pains of ageing have disappeared with Tim's great coaching and teaching.

—Amelia K. (85)

I've worked out and taught fitness classes since I was 18 and I work in PT now, so I know a fair amount about body mechanics. Tim has taught me at a whole other level about the importance of good biomechanics applied to strength training, which has increased my strength like never before, all without injury.

—Lynn F. (60)

Before training with Tim, I'd do the same exercises over and over again with little noticeable improvement. Now with the variety of proper workouts, coupled with the constant attention of Tim to teach and insure proper technique, I have a definite improvement in strength, muscle gain, stamina and feeling good overall.

—Drew F. (61)

I love training with Tim because I'm constantly challenged with new workouts that increase my fitness level. I come from a gymnastics background, so appreciate the methodology and attention to detail in his program. I was looking for more instruction, guidance and results and more is what I got!

—Jill H. (35)

What I've achieved in 2 years has been more than I imagined! I'm feeling better than when I was in college, probably in the best shape of my life and my weight is at an all time low. Weight aside, I'm stronger and more defined than I've ever been. I can't imagine where my body was headed if I hadn't found LifeStrong training.

—Mari W. (49)

Tim's training has been a life-changing experience. Tim said to stick with the program for 90 days and then make an assessment. 18 months later I've lost 35 pounds, reduced my waist size by 3" and decreased my body fat by 8%! At 62 I'm in better shape than in the last 20 years. The program works and it makes it incredibly easy to stay committed when you see the results pile up.

—Chris D. (62)

Prior to this training I had physically plateaued and was feeling uncommitted to any kind of fitness. Thank goodness I found this program-it was exactly what I needed to push and inspire me. I've seen my body literally transform. I've gained muscle and endurance, lost weight and reshaped my body. Beyond the incredible physical benefits, the most monumental piece has been what it's done for me mentally. It has kept me in a healthy routine, boosted my confidence and showed me just how strong I am.

—Emily G. (30)

THE GOAT WITHIN

WITHIN

HEALTHY AND STRONG or SICK AND WEAK?

TIMOTHY J. WARD

AR
PRESS

The GOAT Within: Healthy and Strong or Sick and Weak?

Copyright © 2025 by Timothy J. Ward

The author is not engaged in the practice of medicine, psychology, or any other licensed healthcare profession. The information in this book is provided for educational purposes only and is not intended to serve as a substitute for professional diagnosis, advice, or treatment. Readers should always seek the guidance of a qualified physician, mental health professional, or other licensed provider regarding any questions or concerns about medical or psychological conditions.

All rights reserved. No part of this publication may be reproduced, distributed, or transmitted in any form or by any means, including photocopying, recording, or other electronic or mechanical methods, without the prior written permission of the author, except in the case of brief quotations embodied in critical reviews and certain other noncommercial uses permitted by copyright law. Please do not participate in or encourage piracy of copyrighted materials in violation of the author's rights.

No part of this book may be used for the training of artificial systems, including systems based on artificial intelligence (AI), without the copyright owner's prior permission. This prohibition shall be in force even on platforms and systems that claim to have such rights based on an implied contract for hosting the book.

Library of Congress Control Number: 2025919972

Paperback ISBN: 978-1-969063-07-7
Hardcover ISBN: 978-1-969063-08-4

1. Main category—Nonfiction › Health, Fitness & Dieting › Personal Health › Healthy Living
2. Other category—Nonfiction › Health, Fitness & Dieting › Personal Health › Longevity
3. Other category—Nonfiction › Self-Help › Personal Transformation

AR
PRESS

Published by American Real Publishing
americanrealpublishing.com

TABLE OF CONTENTS

FOREWORD

As a Doctor of Dental Medicine with advanced training in full-mouth rehabilitation and complex cosmetic reconstruction, I've spent years mastering precision, biomechanics, and the intricate anatomy of the human face and jaw. My education demanded complete attention to detail, evidence-based decision-making, and a deep understanding of how every system of the body interconnects. That's why, when it comes to my own health and longevity, I don't leave anything to guesswork or gimmicks.

I found Timothy Ward—and The FITNESS QUADRANT™—when I was searching for a system as refined, detailed, and scientifically grounded as my own professional discipline. What I discovered was something rare in the fitness world: a structured, science-backed method that reflects the same level of rigor I apply to my surgical practice.

The GOAT Within isn't just a book—it's a masterclass in intelligent human performance. Tim has created a fitness ecosystem that rivals medical protocol in its clarity, purpose, and effectiveness. The FITNESS QUADRANT—centered on resistance training, cardiovascular development, strategic nutrition, and recovery—is built on decades of research, yet it's delivered in a way that's clear, practical, and immediately impactful.

Working with Tim has completely changed the way I train, eat, and recover. His protocols are precise—down to the movement pattern, the rest interval, the nutrient timing. His understanding of the human body, from mitochondria to mindset, is nothing short of elite. Just as every millimeter matters in cosmetic reconstruction, every decision matters in fitness after 40. Tim gets that.

This book will open your eyes to what real fitness looks like, including:

Why muscle preservation isn't a vanity metric—it's a major longevity marker and neurological necessity.

Why cardiovascular strength is a powerful predictor of lifespan and how to train it efficiently.

How metabolic health is a critical support system that adequate nutrition fuels.

Why most people are aging faster than they should and how to reverse that decline through a combination of properly targeted strategies and sustainable actions.

And most importantly, how to build a body that triggers all sorts of internal growth metrics, not just one that looks good.

Thanks to Tim's system, I've gained lean muscle, improved flexibility, eliminated chronic aches, and built the kind of strength that carries over into every part of my life—including long clinical days and the sports I love. My energy, clarity, and resilience have all gone to another level.

If you're holding *The GOAT Within*, you're not just holding another fitness book. You're holding a system of principles that, when applied, will radically elevate your physical capacity and slow down the biological aging process.

I've lived it. I've studied it. And I have greatly benefited from it.

—Dr. Tarek Shaib, DMD
Cosmetic and Reconstructive Dentist | Surgical Artist
Advocate for Strength and Longevity | LifeStrong Client

A SPECIAL MESSAGE FROM MY WIFE

I want to share a piece of my journey with you, especially if you're a woman in your 50s or 60s wondering what's still possible for your health.

At 62 years old, I'm 5'5", 125 pounds, and close to as muscular and vibrant as I was in my 30s. Resistance training and nutrition done correctly have been my secret weapons—the anchor through the decades that continues to bless me in ways I never imagined when I first picked up a dumbbell.

When I was younger, lifting weights gave shape to my thin frame and taught me to fuel my body properly. But now, in this season of life, its impact is so much deeper than I realized 30 years ago. Strength, energy, balance, resilience—these are the huge dividends I'm cashing in on today. Weight training has allowed me to twist away from the typical decline of aging: weakness, stiffness, instability, and sickness! I want to run, climb, lift, and play, not struggle with stairs or rising from a chair.

Ladies, I need you to hear this: building strength will not make you "too bulky" or "too masculine." Those are myths. The truth is that resistance training helps prevent falls, protects your bones from osteoporosis, and keeps you feeling confident, capable, and free. Even simple bodyweight exercises can spark powerful changes. What you need is the *right knowledge*—the kind that this book and the Fitness Quadrant system gives you—to stay safe and make the most of your effort.

One of the greatest blessings of my life has been walking this journey side by side with Tim. For 30 years we've made fitness and healthy living a team sport, training together, cooking together, and passing this lifestyle on to our two sons who also work out and have awesome nutrition habits.

My hope is that this legacy carries into future generations and, through this book, into your life as well.

The truth is simple: knowledge + action = power. With the right guidance, you *can* stay strong, avoid injuries, and squeeze every ounce of joy and quality out of life.

If I can do this in my 60s, so can you. Start now, wherever you are, and don't look back. The GOAT within you is waiting.

With love, strength, and encouragement,

Julie

A HEALTHY PERSON WANTS TO DO 1,000 THINGS

A SICK PERSON ONLY WANTS TO DO ONE

Everything seems important until you become sick and/or disabled. At that moment, you realize the only thing that matters is your health. If the richest person in the world was diagnosed with a terminal disease, like stage 4 cancer, severe heart disease, or Alzheimer's, I would bet they would give up their fortune to become 100% cured and return to being healthy and strong.

Health is the most valuable asset in the world. Yet it is rarely prioritized or acted upon preemptively, sad to say, until it is often too late. When you have your health, you don't just have more time, but more quality time. Don't wait until you become too sick and too far gone into decay to realize this. Be preemptive and learn to dramatically tilt the scales of strength and longevity in your favor. Healthier is always happier.

INTRODUCTION

Our lives are a series of many different stories. Our love story. Our financial story. Our success story. Our faith story. Our legacy story. Our childhood story. Our parenting story. Our career story. Our health and wellness story. Our longevity story.

Every story has three major players in it: A villain, a hero, and a guide.

When it comes to your health, wellness, and longevity story, there are actually three main villains for you and most people over 45, which are 1) lack of knowledge, 2) toxic foods, and 3) aging. These three villains prematurely rob most people of their health and longevity.

I am your expert guide who will help you become the hero of your personal health story by giving you the proper fitness and longevity knowledge to defeat the three villains that are already affecting your health.

Make your health and longevity story end with greatness.

Welcome to *The GOAT Within.*

The second we're born, the very first concern from Mom and Dad is to know if the baby is healthy. Does it have all ten toes and ten fingers, and is it vibrant, pink, and screaming? At the other end of life, perhaps our 70s, 80s, and maybe 90s, the same concern begins all over again but from a dramatically opposing viewpoint. Our concerned loved ones, those who are closest to us, say things like, "How is their health?" "Is he or she okay?" "They can't remember where they are supposed to be." "They look so weak and frail." "They can't remember my name anymore."

But what about the part of life between birth and death? This middle part of our journey can extend our life span with strength and purpose by years or accelerate it toward the final hours of our life prematurely, stealing precious years. But what does this middle part look like for most people? What does it look like for you?

This book is about that middle part, *your* middle part. It's about you breaking out of the norm and becoming much more aware and knowledgeable about how to become incredibly fit, healthy, strong, and unstoppable at any age with the help of the principles and lessons within these pages. It's about you living stronger by gaining muscle, strength, and mobility; increasing longevity, decreasing fat stores; and becoming healthier and happier during your personal life journey.

How, you ask? By learning the truth about how to trigger a physical *growth* mode using the four phases of fitness while simultaneously learning how to avoid plunging into a *decay* mode as you age. It is vital to know this, especially if you are 45 or older—an age range when decay mode automatically begins to activate, and even worse, to accelerate at a pace you cannot stop. That is, unless you know how to become a more muscular, flexible, energized fat-burning machine instead of a stiff, tight fat-storage machine. Storing excessive fat invites all sorts of health problems into your life storyline. If you don't know it, I sincerely hope you learn it because there is a cost for everything, and the cost for not understanding this is one you do *not* want to pay. Unfortunately, 90% of Americans will pay the price of decay. Remember, if you are a 38-year-old male or a 40-year-old female, your life is statistically half over. I want to help you change this equation. The question is—are you ready to learn how to become unstoppable?

I have never met a person who is sick and weak and also satisfied, content, and happy.

The human body is a masterpiece of godly engineering, a divine symphony of atoms, DNA, RNA, and living, moving, electrically charged adaptive tissue. It's the ultimate machine, brimming with limitless potential, both physically and mentally. However, this godly machine of yours cannot operate at an optimal level if it is constantly being pumped full of toxic foods and materials, no matter how hard you work at your fitness and wellness. This will be your first lesson.

Just imagine for a moment that you own your dream car, a car you've always wanted. Say it's a European masterpiece—an Aston Martin or McClaren or Ferrari or Porsche 918. The engineering, craftsmanship, and performance are legendary on such machines, as most people know. Imagine, then, that you put contaminated gas in it. This super car would barely start up, barely drive. All that incredible potential would not function properly. What a tragedy to have it all spoiled by bad fuel. The same is true for your body. Bad, toxic foods—your body's fuel and repair components—will ruin its functionality, health, and longevity, especially over time. The very first lessons in Section 1 and Section 2 are focused on identifying the major things pushing your health and longevity backwards. It involves identifying and avoiding toxic nutrition and toxic products that are stealing your future. Only then can you begin laying the foundation for mind-blowing acceleration into physical growth and personal abundance at any age.

The *GOAT Within* highlights your hidden power—especially as you age—to choose a legitimate winning pathway that unlocks it and stimulates growth. This will help you become healthier and stronger, rather than existing in societal norms that *will* make you automatically nosedive into decay, making you sick and weak. Our best choices are always informed ones. They help us carve out a personal path to happiness at a much higher rate compared to going along with uninformed societal norms that are loaded with traps and misinformation that lead to ill-fated conclusions. It's up to you. Pay attention. Nobody is coming to help you. It takes knowledge and consistency to live healthy and strong, and unless these requirements are met, you and your family will suffer the painful consequences of sickness and weakness. Unfortunately, the wellness and fitness space is littered with misinformation and misleading advice. Just look at the statistics—the US is nosediving more than ever into poor health and decay. People need help.

Too many uniformed people suffer premature physical decline and decay because they are distracted and trapped by misinformation. Delusional health and fitness routines and fake nutrition move them *away* from being healthy and strong—away from happiness and satisfaction. Are you one of them? I've witnessed the decline in most people for thirty years now, watching thousands of them inside fitness centers wasting time, getting nowhere. And people outside the gym? Forget about it. It's ugly. Virtually every day, I observe and converse with people and "trainers" inside and outside fitness centers where I work with individuals, groups, and athletic teams. I am right in the thick of it every day, and I see the reality of where people truly are in their health story.

Section 1 will open the doors to the importance of fitness and health knowledge and the consequences of a lack of knowledge. I present some statistics and graphs that demonstrate the actual never-ending fitness struggle and trajectory of the current status quo. Section 1 will also introduce our internal case study story of Skinny Jimmy—a client's journey through our systems from beginning to now in 2025. Section 2 will give a more detailed overview of the toxic environment we must learn to navigate. Learn this part, and you're on the launching pad to incredible health—better than you ever imagined, especially when you add in Section 3: Living Stronger, Better, and Longer.

Successful people are masters at eliminating all sorts of problems. Being *preemptive* is always the best position, and it's a word we use a lot. But when it comes to being fit, strong, and healthy, a vast majority of even the smartest and most accomplished individuals in our society—people who you would expect to prioritize their greatest asset and have a knowledgeable and successful approach to health and wellness—suffer greatly from their declining health and unrealized wellness goals. A vast majority end up in a state of decline and decay as the years go by, and they really don't know why or how. Then, out of the blue, they take a turn for the worse that they never saw coming. A stroke. A slip and fall/broken hip. Sarcopenia (muscle and strength loss). Early dementia. In a majority of the more extreme cases, it's too late to reverse the damage. There are many reasons for this. However, most people do have time to reverse it. But the clock is ticking. If only they had invested as much care and attention into their health and vitality over the past thirty-plus years as they did into their careers and 401(k). Imagine the difference if they'd been *preemptive*. Yes, there's that word again. Section 3 will begin to deliver your solutions and outline some action plans for you.

At some point in your life, fitness, health, and wellness will demand your full attention—by choice or by consequence. Don't wait for a crisis to force your hand. Take control now, before your body makes the decision for you. One of the major problems is that there is no curriculum in schools anywhere in the US that teaches the importance of proper nutrition and fitness. Zero. What has been engineered isn't just millions of dangerously uneducated future generations—it's an army of lifelong addicts hooked on fake, processed food, funneled straight into early sickness, primed to become the perfect cash cows for Big Pharma's never-ending profit train. What a shame.

Here are the three major longevity markers that determine not just how long you live but the quality of your life—stronger, sharper, and with unshakable vitality. You need to put these three things on your radar screen, and if you already know about them, you need to start an adequate program that will strengthen each one if you truly want to extend your life with quality living.

Muscle Mass and Strength – your body's armor against aging.

Cardiovascular Strength – the engine that keeps your heart, brain, and stamina alive.

Metabolic Health – staying insulin sensitive, not insulin resistive, through proper nutrition to avoid the slow decay caused by modern disease.

These aren't just health stats—they're your *lifelines*. And the key to optimizing all three? Our proven, trademarked system that addresses all three and more: The FITNESS QUADRANT™. It's the ultimate blueprint for building a body and a personal health ecosystem that resists aging, disease, and decline. Follow it—and add years to your life and life to your years.

During the last thirty-five years, I have had the privilege of integrating myself with some of the best exercise scientists and researchers in the world. I've been exposed to premium life-changing data along with coaching hundreds of clients and athletes through various levels of science-based protocols. I have been very fortunate to have gained the ability to translate real exercise science and data into unique transformative fitness routines and nutrition systems that produce massive results for people of all ages. From being hands-on through thousands of workouts and countless personal success stories, I have seen what works and what doesn't. I am an expert trainer and longevity coach who has been the guy on the floor, perfecting my craft into highly effective, achievable, and sustainable systems.

The information and systems described in this book and the real-time experiences I have had with so many people have changed many lives for the better. The people that have learned and adopted the methods in our FITNESS QUADRANT system have hit what we call fitness momentum. It's a point where everything comes together after about eight to twelve weeks and then starts to exponentially grab hold. It's a feeling that's indescribable. Healthy and strong—finally! I am honored and blessed to share some of this vital information with you. Oh, and guess what? Willpower alone will not give you better results if you lack the real knowledge to train properly—I don't care who you are. In fact, willpower coupled with incorrect biomechanics (exercise form) and poor training habits will get you injured much more quickly, which defeats the whole purpose, no? I've witnessed willpower wreck many people with bad injuries over the years.

I always tell people, "Do your own research and see what you come up with." You'll uncover a mountain range of deep science that will most likely give you a headache, and you'll soon realize just how complex the human body is when it comes to proper fitness practices.

The marketplace of wellness and fitness is littered with misinformation. I am not a famous Hollywood doctor or celebrity who is leveraging my fame to make millions of dollars by hiring ghostwriting teams and expensive publishing houses to capitalize on my fame by marketing a book with the primary goal of generating more money for myself. This book is about the real stuff that will apply to you. I am the creator and coach. Unlike the famous docs and celebrities, I am not attempting to game the fitness and wellness space. The principles in this book have generated real results for an array of my clients—ranging from young and athletic people to older men and women in their 70s and 80s who were looking to bring back some strength and mobility so they could squeeze out some last active years of their lives. I built Modified Interval Training™ (MIT) and The FITNESS QUADRANT for people who don't want to attempt to go through painstaking years of *trying* to figure this stuff out. Chances are, you won't—no offense. There is simply too much specialized knowledge and information that exists. It has all come together for me at the right times and circumstances in my life with the right people. Not to mention my many years in fierce pursuit of higher understanding.

Since the early 2000s, many of my friends and family, frustrated with their fitness results or just plain lost when they tried to work out or eat better, have asked me to help them with their exercise routines and nutrition. I have happily written so many plans for them through the years that I've lost count. The impetus for this book was to pull together something more formal that might be read by enough people that it might make a difference to a handful of them.

There are major takeaways for you that are woven into this book. They are the very reason I pursued it, as challenging as it was for me. These takeaways are very substantial when it comes to achieving actual success with your health and well-being. The most profound overarching lesson is that your path to superior success is rooted in the four different phases of fitness, which you will learn about in The FITNESS QUADRANT. The combination of these four quadrants will give you access to huge success, at any age or level of fitness. I cannot overstate enough the fact that there is an appropriate entry point for everyone when it comes to either starting or refining your weekly fitness and wellness routine. Unlike the famous Hollywood doctors and actors who *produce* heavily marketed 400-page books about stats and complex research articles on fitness and longevity, *I'm the experienced and educated guy on the ground doing the actual work* with hundreds of people every year—including many doctors, by the way—educating them on properly sequenced workouts, exercise form, and selection. The nutrition and cardio protocols, mobility and recovery plans I design for them are taking off that 30+ pounds *of fat* while dramatically *increasing their muscle mass and mobility*, fixing sore knees, shoulders, correcting posture and ailing lower backs, making them happier and their lives better.

You see, I too, at the age of 60, am a lifelong athlete who has always kept in shape and always participated in various sports, including basketball, football, baseball, tennis, golf, jiu-jitsu, and other martial arts. I too have had to modify my approach as I age. There came a point when I was in my late 20s when I knew my fitness routine wasn't up to par. I went wandering into the gym three days a week picking exercises at random, then doing them with poor biomechanics and no direction. Most importantly, I was seeing minimal changes to my body no matter how hard I tried.

It was then that I met and trained for four years with an exercise scientist who opened the door for me into a world of in-depth research on exercise. It changed my trajectory and set me on a very aggressive path to further educate myself and get linked into the PhD research that sifts out the garbage and myths and proves theories through extensive complex studies and experimentation. *The real stuff.* I took courses and got various certifications, which, by the way, are mostly window dressing and are largely insufficient for what you need to transform lives or write appropriate training protocols that address the performance needs of top-level athletes or solve problems of everyday people looking to get in shape at their local gym or at home. This is part of the problem in the fitness space.

In an odd way, I salute most of these mega-popular Hollywood doctors and celebrities who have at least brought attention to the importance of fitness, longevity, and wellness. That's a good thing. However, I would challenge any of them at any time to write a fitness and longevity protocol that could compete with my systems. Best of luck to them. My priority is to give you practical, unique, and usable information, not to sell millions of books by simply citing research studies, which seems to be *their PR handlers'* priority. Although, selling a million books would be kind of nice.

I've got you. Let's roll.

CONNECT AND LEARN WITH US:

www.fitnessquadrant.net

www.skool.com/lifestrong/about

LINKEDIN: linkedin.com/in/coach-timothy-ward

INSTAGRAM: FITNESSQUADRANT

Living things move.
Dead things do not move.

At any age, and only under certain
conditions,
muscle grows, fat burns,
heart and lungs strengthen,
joints get lubricated and smooth,
balance and stability are restored,
metabolism stabilizes,
energy levels go through the roof,
and you rise up to healthy and happy.

Or, under certain other conditions,
you lose muscle, you gain fat,
heart and lungs weaken,
joints seize up,
you lose balance and stability,
metabolism sinks,
energy levels dry up,
and you accelerate into decay.

SECTION 1

SHEER MADNESS

Over the last fifteen years, we have seen an increase in gym-goers by tracking membership growth statistics in the US. But hold on a minute. The harsh reality is that all the health-related sicknesses, obesity rates, and diseases are piling up and rising faster than gym memberships! How is that possible? More gym memberships than ever, yet more people than ever are diving into decay and sickness? What is behind this fitness dilemma?

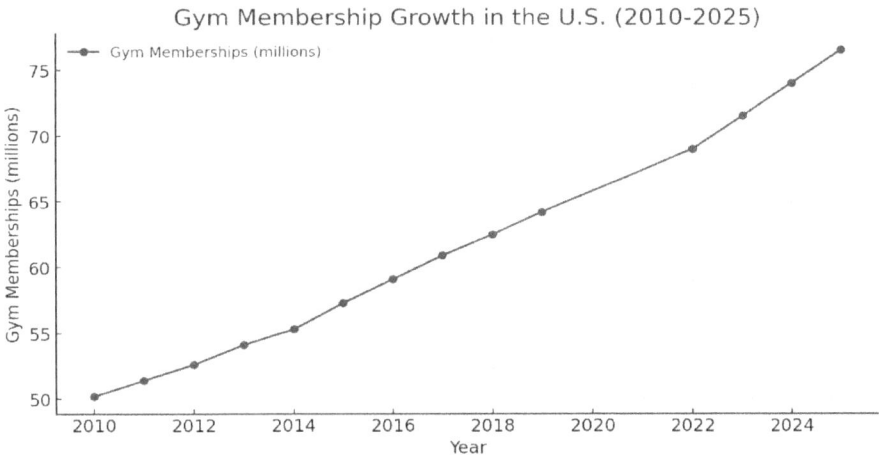

Gym Membership Growth in the U.S. (2010-2025)

Despite an increase from approximately 50.2 million memberships in 2010 to approximately 78 million in 2025, America has grown sicker than ever during this period. The logic doesn't make sense. However, there is a distinct reason for this. Population growth plays a small role, but inadequate fitness practices and a toxic food environment are the real culprits.

As a whole, a severe lack of fitness and health knowledge is fueling these losing outcomes.

CHAPTER 1

WHAT DOES YOUR LIFE CURVE LOOK LIKE?

THE BLACK DOG

The black dog is everything that's destructive in your life. It will devour you. This is decay.

Sedentary lifestyle, narcissism, anger, hate, fake and phony, revengeful, bitterness, lying, two-faced, deceptive, cheating, stealing, dishonesty, disingenuousness, untrustworthiness, being short-fused, hot tempered, arrogance, self-centeredness, cheapness, being unfriendly and unkind, alcohol abuse, drug abuse, being non-charitable, unreliable, a manipulator, two-faced, greedy, blaming others, self-righteous, self-promotion, and living a toxic anti-health lifestyle.

THE WHITE DOG

The white dog is everything positive in your life. It will empower you. This is growth.

Truthfulness, godliness, being family-centered, courageous, thankful, grateful, graceful, loving, trustworthy, compassionate, humble, giving, honest, health-focused, hardworking, committed, selfless, calm, approachable, solution oriented, introspective, a goal setter, following through, and helping others.

Which dog have you been feeding lately?

Will you live on to be healthy and strong, or will you become sick and weak and have your life curve prematurely shortened? Healthy and strong is so attainable to the vast majority. It's literally a matter of having the desire and courage to decide to pursue correct knowledge, taking action, and staying consistent. You can change the trajectory of your life.

Growth: Healthy & Strong

High

Quality
of Life

Average

Low

Decay: Sick & Weak

Birth

Death

0   10   20   30   40   50   60   70   80   90   100

Age

LIFE STRONG
HEALTHIER IS HAPPIER

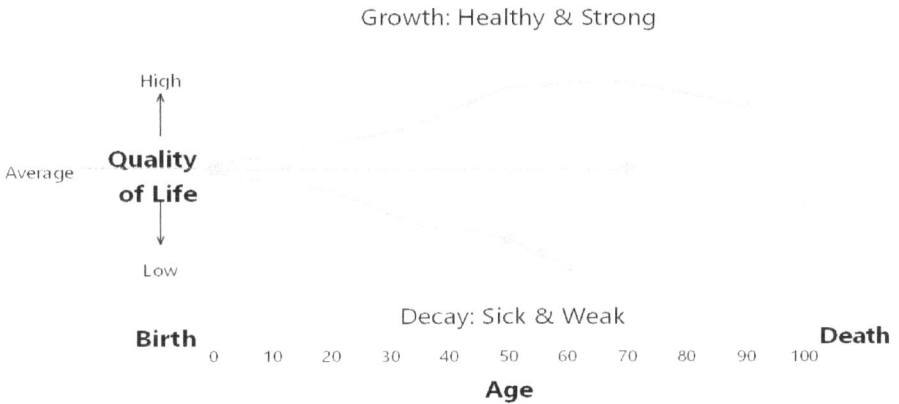

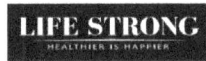

The seeds of health, vitality, high energy, longevity, and happiness lie in our grasp, closer than we can ever imagine. The answers are right in front of us yet remain so elusive to the masses. Our society has become distracted with misinformation and mindless habits (excessive drinking, binge watching Netflix series, and social media scrolling ring a bell?) that hold our attention for hours every day. They steal our focus away from spending time on real issues that are dramatically vital to our survival and well-being.

If there was a super health pill—one that embodied all the accurate science, all the perfect mechanisms of living a strong, vibrant, healthy life, void of toxic micro-ingredients and harmful side effects—it would be worth trillions of dollars. There would be billions of customers, and it would be hailed as one of the greatest discoveries in the history of mankind. Instead, $4+ trillion per year is spent on medical and hospital care and pharmaceuticals, not to cure but rather to *manage* problems of diseases and sicknesses that could otherwise be virtually mitigated with proper knowledge and responsible food production practices. This multitrillion-dollar sickness management model is not a mistake, by the way. It's one of the biggest money trains on the planet—big, powerful, and massively profitable.

That magic pill doesn't exist, as we all know. But what does exist is a magic formula and an abundance of proven pathways that will get you very far down the road to health, longevity, and wellness. When you look at these individual pieces and get to a point where you understand them and how they fit together, you'll get closer and closer to accessing the greatness that lies within you—THE GOAT WITHIN. Consider these pieces as different sets of keys that when put together can unlock multiple vital doors to increased health, strength, and longevity that are otherwise closed and inaccessible because of misinformation and lack of knowledge.

The path to living healthy and strong is not one dimensional. It is *multiple pieces* that work synergistically in combination and allow you to elevate your game to achieve high levels of health and vitality and push you into strength and longevity. The greatest workouts in the world are brought to their knees and rendered useless when we practice poor nutrition and lifestyle habits. Our toxic world is so sneaky and disguised. Mass toxicity can be found in virtually every part of our lives, from mass-produced toxic food and materials we touch and use every day to our tainted water supply. It's all literally unavoidable if you lack the knowledge or are not well informed enough. And eating a healthy diet alone will not drive your health and longevity to the heights it could reach unless you're adding in proper strength and muscle-building protocols that trigger the body to use those nutritional substrates at a much higher rate. *In combination, all the right pieces enhance each other*. You must have multiple components that are connected in order to succeed. These are the *four phases* to healthy and strong. This is at the very core of The FITNESS QUADRANT™ system. It's your personalized master blueprint to build your longevity and wellness ecosystem.

FOUR LEVELS
OF COMPETENCY

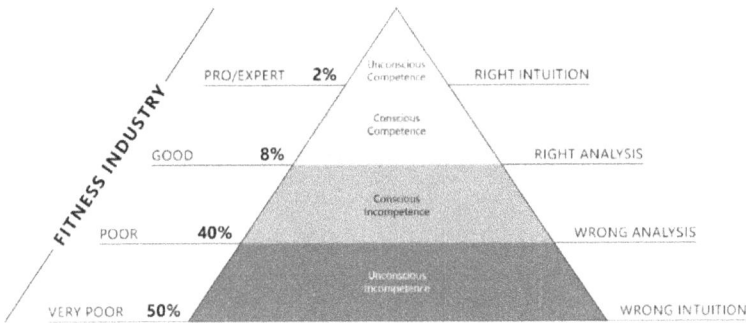

FITNESS INDUSTRY				
PRO/EXPERT	2%	Unconscious Competence	RIGHT INTUITION
		Conscious Competence	
GOOD	8%		RIGHT ANALYSIS
		Conscious Incompetence	
POOR	40%		WRONG ANALYSIS
		Unconscious Incompetence	
VERY POOR	50%		WRONG INTUITION

LIFE STRONG
HEALTHIER IS HAPPIER

You don't know what you don't know, as depicted in the bottom two levels of the competency triangle above, which literally make up 90% of the fitness sector. It's not their fault—they have never been exposed to scientific methods of fitness. They're simply blind and suffer from unconscious and conscious incompetence.

There is no other industry that is so open-ended, where you can take something as complex as the human body and have at it with commercial fitness machinery and equipment for $10 per month. Such equipment can seriously hurt you when used incorrectly (which happens 90% of the time), leading to things like torn rotator cuffs (shoulders), injured lower backs, sore knee joints, strained hamstrings, etc., all while people think they are getting fit and in shape.

Fitness is one of the few industries that often delivers zero returns to about 90% of its participants, and yet the same people repeat the same "workout" every week.

Would you be happy if your 401k delivered 0% year after year?

You'd probably look for a different strategy.

FAKE FOOD, FAKE FITNESS, AND PHARMACEUTICALS

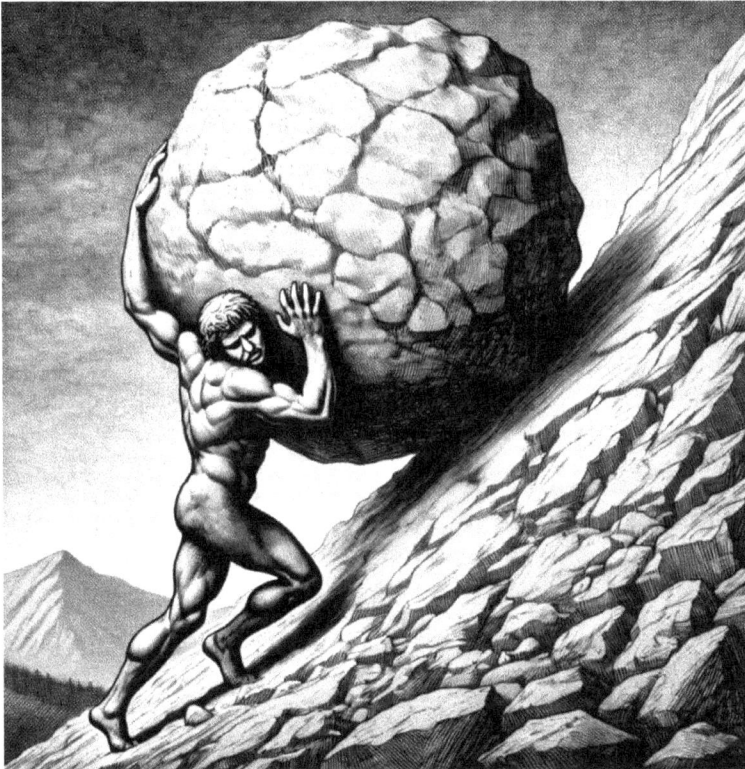

THE SISYPHEAN STRUGGLE AND FITNESS FRUSTRATION

In Greek mythology, Sisyphus was condemned to push a massive boulder up a hill for eternity, only for it to roll back down each time he neared the summit. His struggle was one of endless effort without reward—a fitting metaphor for the modern fitness industry, where millions battle to lose weight and build muscle but ultimately fail over and over again.

Every year, nearly 100 million people embark on fitness journeys with high hopes, only to fall short of their goals. They lift, run, diet, and sweat, but the results never match the effort. Why? Because they're trapped in a cycle of misinformation, ineffective training, and injury setbacks—a Sisyphean cycle where they push forward only to slide back down.

The Core Issues Behind Fitness Failure

1. Fake Fitness and Fake Food – The fitness industry sadly thrives on quick fixes, fad diets, and ineffective programs that lead people astray. Without understanding the right way to exercise at the appropriate level and how to avoid toxic fake food and replace it with adequate proper nutrition, most waste years on flawed methods.

2. Injury and Setbacks – Strength training without proper mechanics leads to ineffective results and chronic pain, injuries, and forced inactivity. Many quit entirely, seeing fitness as an uphill battle they'll never win.

3. Inefficient Workouts – Most people undertrain, overtrain, or follow inadequate cookie-cutter routines that don't align with their needs or are severely incorrect in their exercise selections. They work hard but not smart, leading to burnout with little progress.

4. Aging and Recovery Limitations – As people hit their 50s and beyond, the old-school "No pain, no gain" mindset fails them. Their bodies demand precision and proper scientific protocols, not punishment.

5. The Doc's Prescription – Of course, there is a pharmaceutical for everything under the sun. This rarely fixes the problem but simply manages it and often causes imbalances in your body that lead to more prescriptions. It just never ends.

Breaking Free from the Cycle

Just as Sisyphus was doomed by fate, most gym-goers feel doomed by their own physiology. But the truth is, the right system can break the cycle. The FITNESS QUADRANT system described in Section 3 provides a structured, science-backed approach to building strength, endurance, mobility, and metabolic health without the frustration and setbacks. Instead of rolling the boulder endlessly, it's time to find a smarter way to reach the summit—and stay there.

THE NEXT "NEW" MIRACLE FITNESS PRODUCT

Our society's desperation for thinness causes a relentless pursuit of weight loss—thus triggering a goldrush for thousands of deceptive companies peddling everything from creams and supplements to meal plans and fitness gadgets claiming to aid in this goal. Each product is marketed as the next "miracle" solution, promising to transform an overweight, out-of-shape body into peak physical condition. With a constant flood of new programs and devices, consumers are led to believe the next one will finally work—only to be met with disappointment after wasting time, money, and hope. Companies with big marketing budgets enjoy their brief moment of fame before fading into obscurity with packed pockets while disillusioned buyers continue searching for the next quick fix or give up entirely.

Now, imagine you're one of the millions desperate for change. You come across yet another product boasting guaranteed weight loss, improved body composition, boundless energy, all-natural ingredients, no side effects, and scientific backing. It sounds too good to be true—because it is. Yet many will still hand over their credit cards while the FTC scrambles to remove yet another false-advertising scam from the airwaves. Nothing but gimmicks, over and over again. Talk about a Sisyphean struggle.

THE TWO FACES OF FREEDOM

Freedom in the Human Spirit

Freedom is the lifeblood of the human soul. Without it, we shrink. With it, we soar. History has shown us in brutal detail what happens when men and women are stripped of their God-given right to live freely. Look at the citizens of suppressed communist-ruled nations—China, Venezuela, Cuba. These are societies where individuality is crushed beneath the weight of the collective, where personal ambition is not celebrated but punished, where voices are silenced, and lives are lived in quiet desperation. In these environments, growth is forbidden, curiosity is dangerous, and independence is outlawed. The result is misery. Depravity. A hollow existence where people survive, but they do not truly live.

Freedom, then, is more than a political idea. It is a psychological necessity to our spirit. When you take away a person's freedom, you take away their ability to think for themselves, to grow, to rise into their potential. They become caged—alive in body but enslaved in mind. And nothing is more corrosive to the human spirit than to be trapped with no chance of escape, no chance to find their GOAT within.

The Freedom Within

But here's the truth most people miss: oppression doesn't only come from governments or dictators. It exists in our modern world in a quieter, more sinister form. The poisons of mass-produced foods, the endless stream of toxic household products, endless pharmaceutical prescriptions, the engineered addictions of sugar, processed seed oils, trans fats, and chemicals—they chain us. They weaken us. They make us sick, tired, foggy, and dependent. They rob us of the most important freedom of all: *the freedom over our own bodies.* And all of this they make seem normal through fake media advertising and news coverage.

This is where building your personal The Fitness Quadrant™ ecosystem becomes your key to physical and mental liberation. True personal freedom is not just about speech or borders—it's about reclaiming your physical and mental sovereignty. By following the protocols of resistance training, cardiovascular conditioning, proper nutrition, and intelligent recovery, you begin to break free from the invisible prison of toxicity and decay. You build muscle—your shield against aging. You sharpen your mind with vitality and energy. You move with strength, power, and mobility, no longer limited by stiffness, fatigue, or unnecessary vaccines, endless pharmaceuticals and man-made diseases.

This is the kind of freedom you can control. Freedom to wake up energized. Freedom to move without pain. Freedom to live on your own terms instead of being shackled by the consequences of our toxic world. And unlike the external freedoms of nations and politics, this freedom is yours for the taking. No government can give it to you, and no dictator can take it away. It lives inside you, waiting to be unlocked.

Freedom is strength. Freedom is health. Freedom is clarity. And the door to that freedom opens when you walk through the Fitness Quadrant and find the GOAT within yourself.

NO EASY WAY TO SAY THIS

Oh, the madness that encapsulates this "fitness" industry. Wow. Multibillion-dollar industries rarely have zero accountability when it comes to the things they supposedly stand for. The fitness industry, however, is the poster child of it. I have never seen such utter chaos as when I've stepped into hundreds of gyms over the years, from New Hampshire to Spain to Portugal to NYC to Miami to Vegas to Boston and LA.

The industry is loaded to the hilt with fake fitness practices and gadgets. Delusional. Full of myths mostly spread by companies and sleazy businesspeople that prey on consumers' emotional pain points with garbage products. Then there are the incompetent gym rats and unknowing trainers who "just got their certification this weekend." They offer false advertising, incorrect exercises, incorrect patterns, incorrect timing, and incorrect advice. These unqualified people are not just incompetent—their advice often leads to injury-inducing movements. I see it over and over again on a daily basis. Don't get me wrong here. I tip my hat to all the people who are actually trying to get fit and get into an effective routine that they think will have some sort of positive effect. Kudos to all of them. They've got the first part down—showing up. But it's what happens from there that matters. This is the painful part for me, being a witness to all this crazy stuff. Once again, an $80+ billion industry, steeped in chaos and ill-fated protocols for the vast majority of consumers.

And it's no wonder. Just look at the crazy reels on social media including movie and music celebrities and Hollywood doctors who are grossly unqualified to preach proper fitness practices to the masses. But they think their fame or the letters "Dr" in front of their names qualifies them. Nothing could be more enraging to me than seeing the books some of them have written about the topic of fitness and longevity— empty chapters that regurgitate a bunch of "studies" and research, but nothing on actual sound fitness practices. Why is this? Because they never learned a speck of it in medical school. They don't teach exercise physiology or nutrition in the curriculum. They do not know about fitness sciences.

A few of these doctors I have great respect for because they actually admit in their books and social media that people in the traditional medical industry—across the board—are never taught anything about proper exercise or nutrition in medical school. They are taught how to treat and *manage* symptoms and which drugs to prescribe after the fact, instead of learning about preventive solutions and lifestyles to avoid sickness and decay. I have first-hand experience with my own doctor, who is 60 pounds overweight, thinks that playing golf two times per week is a great fitness routine because she doesn't use a cart, she walks the eighteen holes. This is a trillion-dollar problem. *Trillion.* And it's getting worse, not better. Just look at the statistics on the growth of diseases and the robust growth of pharmaceutical companies. It's not hard to figure out what's going on. Wall Street bankers, politicians, and big food manufacturers control the spigot on all of this for two reasons and two reasons only. Profit and power—at your expense. Let that sink in.

And let's not forget misinformation and misleading advice at its finest with the absolutely criminal social media "fitness coaching gurus" who promise to train any and all trainers on their "breakthrough lead-generation system" of how to "make $60,000 per month" with online training for marketing to new clients. These people, usually young punks with tattoos all over them, pushing false promises of riches to unsuspecting and underqualified trainers, actually make the most outrageous claims. They say things like "100% money back guarantee if our revolutionary system doesn't make you $20,000 in your first 30 days!" Then they hit new trainers with a $10,000 sign-up fee and laugh at them when they ask for their money back.

How do I know this? I just tested out one of these real low-life sales groups from Miami, which I will not name. They teach fitness trainers how to pressure sell big ticket fitness programs to the unsuspecting public who are looking to lose weight and get fit. It was the most comical and complete scam I have seen in a while. I posed (and paid a small fee) as a trainer interested in their system. And wow, the promises that were made! They had no idea I was researching these scams for this book. These types of people would take $10,000 from *anyone*, regardless of their fitness background. And believe me, when I saw the "trainers" they were bringing on…WHOA. These people couldn't teach you how to do a squat or push-up the right way. Yet this scam company continues to push—and scam—low-level fitness "trainers" out into the fitness ecosystem and lie to unsuspecting people by selling them false fitness dreams and routines with promises of grandeur. This is a shining example of why the fitness industry needs to be regulated somehow to weed out companies that only have deception and their wallets as a priority. It's disgusting, and the end consumer pays the price and the fitness industry gets a black eye.

CHAPTER 3

THE GIFT
OF CHOICE

One of the most powerful gifts we have been given from God is the power of choice. Clearly, we all know what choosing poorly can mean. These **black dog** choices hurt us, and unfortunately, hurt our loved ones as well. We have all chosen poorly at some point in our lives. If we had the power to go back in time and change some of those decisions, I bet 99% of us would.

On the other side, we have the **white dog** choices. These good choices lift us up, higher and higher, and most of the time they lift other people up around us as well. Keep stringing together good choices and your journey to success and happiness will become more of a reality every day. Now we're talking. The power of choice is the deciding moment of change, either good or bad. Choose wisely. This is where it all begins or ends for you and me. In the spirit of health and longevity, let's choose healthy and strong instead of sick and weak.

The understanding of what living in a *growth* mode is compared to living in a *decay* mode is an undeniable revelation when you grasp it. It is only upon capturing the proper knowledge that one can take proper action—the how-to that will give you all you need to turn on the growth switch. But the journey only succeeds when you decide to implement it. That is the mission of this book: to get you to prioritize your health and well-being.

Four steps to designing your successful strength and longevity ecosystem:

- Knowledge
- Game plan
- Implementation
- Consistency

Why would you trade 100% of your time for work, play, and leisure and not commit 5% of your time to the proper way of achieving fitness, longevity, and badassery? Your health is your greatest asset and will always be your greatest asset. Doesn't it deserve 5% of your weekly time? We're talking about three to four hours per week. Is this reasonable to you? No?

GROWTH OR DECAY

No decision could make as much of an impact on your lifespan—and equally as important, the *quality* of your lifespan—as the decision to live in a *growth* mode, being *healthy and strong*, instead of living in *decay* mode, being *sick and weak*.

You first have to understand this:

GROWTH – you WIN

During an *anabolic state*, metabolic processes in the body *build* and *repair* muscle tissue. The body is in an anabolic state when it's consuming energy to build muscle mass. This is the opposite of a catabolic state, when the body breaks down tissue to replenish energy.

OR

DECAY – you LOSE

A *catabolic state* is a metabolic state where the body breaks down complex molecules and muscle (along with a process called gluconeogenesis) to release energy. This causes you to *lose muscle mass and all your vital internal components slip into decline.*

Understanding what triggers growth is the point, and it is a choice. Our quality of life, wellness, and longevity are directly impacted by our daily choices—except of course for unavoidable circumstances, accidents and/or unfortunate tragedies. One of the cruelest things in humanity is watching the aging process prematurely rob people of their wellness and their ability to be strong, vibrant, healthy, mobile, active, and happy.

In reality, we have the ability to slow down the physical and mental decline that happens with aging. Premature physical decline is brought on and accelerated by a lack of knowledge and lack of action that leads to poor lifestyle choices, which in turn lead us directly into physical decay and unnecessary suffering. It really is all about growth or decay. Growth mode means you place yourself in an anabolic state and decay mode means you place yourself in a catabolic state. Doing nothing or going through the motions of inadequate fitness keeps you in a catabolic state. It truly is a choice that requires knowledge to unpack the differences.

Just showing up to the gym is not
enough to move the needle.

You need knowledge on how to execute
proper fitness protocols and wellness habits.

Superior fitness programs are most definitely
transformational. However, the roadmap to get
there is transactional.

You cannot get to the transformation
without the weekly transactions.

TWO PROFOUND EQUATIONS
YOU MUST UNDERSTAND

DECAY looks like this:

INACTIVITY OR INADEQUATE FITNESS

+

TOXIC OR INADEQUATE NUTRITION

=

DECAY

=

LOWER QUALITY OF LIFE

=

PREMATURE DEATH

GROWTH looks like this:

ADEQUATE FITNESS

+

ADEQUATE NUTRITION

=

GROWTH

=

HIGHER QUALITY OF LIFE

=

LONGEVITY

THE CURRENCIES OF THE HUMAN BODY

We always equate currency with money—US dollars. But the body has a different type of currency.

Imagine for a minute, you have $1 million in your bank account. That's all you have. You cannot put any more in. And let's imagine that you draw on that $1 million for every expense you have for the rest of your life. What do you have left in the account after ten years? How about in twenty years? Maybe $5,000? $0?

Now let's take that $1 million and convert it into 1 million units of your body's physical currency—the vital components that are the currency of vitality, strength, vibrancy, energy, repair, cognitive ability, etc.

As you age, these physical currencies are naturally depleting, and you feel the effects more and more as the years go by. When you understand this, you'll consider an action plan that rebuilds these currencies in your body. Think of this plan as an investment that is giving you an ROI, or return on investment, of 15% per year on your physical currency supply. And FYI—more pharmaceuticals from "the doc" to treat "symptoms" are *not* the answer. They are part of the problem.

When you're young, you have what seems to be an endless stash of this physical currency. It's what keeps you feeling young, strong, and healthy. When you are young, you can also replenish it readily because the internal systems of youth are fully charged and at full production. But once you are about 45 years old, certainly 50+, not only are you unable to effortlessly replace it anymore, but you actually begin to lose these currency units at an accelerated pace. *Especially* when you live in a toxic catabolic environment of poor nutrition and practice a sedentary lifestyle where proper exercise is nonexistent. As the years go on, the rate at which you lose this physical currency speeds up. This will age you faster than time itself and will cripple your quality of life along the way. This is the very reason you need a plan to counteract these losses, to push back on them.

LONGEVITY COMPONENTS

Your body's "currency" that are in decline once you are around **45 years old**. Unfortunately, while you are losing these vital pieces, you are simultaneously increasing the components of DECAY that are aging you faster and faster as the years tick by.

IN DECLINE
Vital pieces you are LOSING as you age:

MUSCLE. A vital marker of your longevity

BONE DENSITY. Onset of frailty and restrictive living

HGH. The fountain of youth hormone

TESTOSTERONE. The alpha male hormone

NITRIC OXIDE. A pivotal compound essential for cardiorespiratory health

GUT BACTERIA. What determines substrate breakdown and usage

STEM CELLS. Cells of youth for repair and vitality

CAPILLARIES. Storage sites of stem cells, blood flow and oxygen

MITOCHONDRIA. Storage and manufacturing organelles of energy and stem cells

SYNOVIAL FLUID. The lubrication substance for joint mobility

ON THE INCREASE
GROWING signs and issues of premature aging:

FAT WEIGHT AND FAT STORAGE. Body fat, visceral, and organ fat

HIGHER BLOOD PRESSURE. Increased BPM

WEAKNESS. Loss of muscle, strength and balance (sarcopenia)

JOINT STIFFNESS. Loss of movement / slip and fall

LOWER ENERGY. Less and less active

LONGER RECOVERY TIME. Loss of time

INJURIES. More susceptible

LESS BODY MOBILITY. Harder to perform normal tasks

WEAKER IMMUNE SYSTEM. Normal illness becomes severe

INSOMNIA / POOR SLEEP. A decline in quality of life

LIFE STRONG
HEALTHIER IS HAPPIER

SARCOPENIA AND FRAILTY

Sarcopenia is a condition of accelerated muscle loss and weakness that triggers frailty. It is brought on by the aging process and accelerated by a lifestyle of living in decay. Sarcopenia can be counteracted and overcome by living in a growth mode. By the time you are 65, you will have a mere 50% left of the very components that keep us youthful. This is not good. This decline (especially muscle loss) is what triggers sarcopenia, which causes frailty. Your best bet is to start with a comprehensive resistance training routine in your early years (30s) and connect it to proper nutritional habits and stick with it for the rest of your life.

Now for some good news. It is *not* too late to start turning on the growth switches again if you are in your 50s, 60s, or 70s. You just need the proper knowledge and guidance.

The following four vital mechanisms—and in certain instances coupled with regenerative tissue therapies (peptides, mesenchymal stem cells and exosomes)—reverse this physical decline and *stimulate the body to trigger the systems of growth* that are otherwise in constant decline as you age. You literally can reverse your decline and take years off your life if you learn to engage in the proper fitness protocols outlined in The FITNESS QUADRANT. And just to note, most fitness routines that are widely practiced every day by millions of people are completely inadequate and will not trigger these systems.

1. *Resistance training

2. *Nutrition and targeted supplementation

3. *Cardiovascular training

4. Peptides: The ultimate new regenerative therapy

*These first three systems are the foundations of triggering growth only when learned properly and then connected with each other. When peptides are added into this equation as super supplements, you rapidly move into what I call your ultimate personal fitness ecosystem.

Through the first three platforms, you can trigger the body internally to dramatically slow the aging process and live a lifestyle of growth (anabolic) into your 70s, 80s, and beyond. The fourth involves peptides as a transformative regenerative therapy. By using external aids to build back reserves of stem cells, testosterone levels, HGH levels, etc., you can dramatically slow aging and reverse the nosedive into decay. *The GOAT Within* gives you the strategies and the wherewithal to offset the decline that so many people prematurely suffer. All three of the first platforms are vital, with resistance training being the holy grail (as you'll see), and it is paramount that it is executed properly. And although not a hard requirement, when you add peptides into this fitness ecosystem, you have built an unstoppable anabolic growth platform for yourself. Just imagine looking, feeling, and moving around like you did fifteen years ago.

Why Peptides and What Are They?

Our clients are experiencing incredible benefits from our peptide protocols.

Peptides are rapidly redefining what's possible in human health and performance. These short chains of amino acids are naturally occurring in your body, but they rapidly decline with age—starting around 45 years old. They act like precision messengers in the body—targeting specific cells and functions to accelerate healing, stimulate growth, and regulate key physiological systems. Though our bodies naturally produce peptides, science has now isolated and refined synthetic versions that can dramatically enhance recovery, muscle development, fat metabolism, and even cognitive performance.

Unlike traditional pharmaceuticals that often have broad, blunt effects, peptides are highly targeted and biologically compatible, making them a breakthrough tool in modern therapeutic protocols.

As an example, these two particular peptides we work with (and dozens more) are revolutionizing the fields of longevity and body optimization. CJC-1295 is a growth hormone-releasing hormone analog that promotes the body's own production of growth hormone—supporting lean muscle growth, fat burning, improved sleep, and anti-aging benefits without the risks of synthetic hormone replacement. BPC-157, often called the "Wolverine peptide," is derived from a protective protein in the stomach and is renowned for its ability to accelerate healing of muscles, tendons, joints, and even gut tissue. Both of these compounds are at the forefront of a new era—where smart biological therapies can extend quality of life, restore damaged tissue, and elevate human potential far beyond what was previously thought possible. It is truly an exciting time to have these next-level therapeutic options that are directly impacting all of us in our 50s and beyond.

LET'S PUT SOME CURRENCY BACK INTO YOUR BANK

Alright, are you ready to get into a growth mode? Let me tell you something. As you age, it's not only possible but also proven that you can turn on the metabolic triggers that actually start putting physical currency—your "physical money"—back into your body's bank account. This means more muscle, more energy, higher metabolism, more activities, more memories. Start the engines up and start to rebuild the factors that you are losing with age, changing inadequate fitness practices and toxic nutrition and lifestyle choices. It will take knowledge, planning, action, and time, but it's a worthwhile, life-changing endeavor indeed.

THE EVOLUTION OF HEALTH AND FITNESS

Some of us remember or have seen old footage of Jack LaLanne or Reg Park in the 50s and 60s, or even Jane Fonda in the 80s. It was impressive to see the "strongmen" and "aerobic queens" of those periods and all of their stunts and showmanship. And who could forget Richard Simmons? Now, seventy years later, today's super athletes, strongmen, and fitness regimens are truly at levels that Jack LaLanne couldn't have imagined. The chronology and definition of "athlete" or what it means to be strong has changed dramatically over those seven decades. Just look at today's examples—Giannis Antetokounmpo, Georges St-Pierre, or Joe Rogan, who is famous for his podcast but also his fitness level and his martial arts and jiu-jitsu background. It's not even comparable. How come?

It comes down to a dramatic increase in the use of technology and scientific studies on human performance in a cross-section of fields ranging from exercise kinesiology—strength and cardiorespiratory—nutrition, athletic performance, aging and gerontology, regenerative medicine, neuroscience, etc.

Today, fitness is different than it was in the 70s, 80s, 90s, and early 2000s, yet you see a lot of the same stuff in gyms across America: a virtual complete lack of knowledge. It's only in professional sports or Olympic training centers that you'll find cutting-edge, science-based fitness practices. This is where the PhDs of the world get to implement their studies. The good stuff rarely makes it down into society.

When modern fitness sciences are employed into structured weekly programs for a vast majority of society, the results can be staggering for a very wide swath of everyday people, not just professional athletes who we already know get top-notch coaching.

MY CLIENTS ARE THRIVING

I have put these growth components in place (see the description of The FITNESS QUADRANT in Section 3) for countless clients in the past and present, and the greatest part of my journey is always watching the transformation that takes place with them. It's awesome and so satisfying to see them learn, commit, and change. The majority of them are 40 to 84 years old (with the exception of my younger athletes), and before they became my clients, they all had one thing in common:

> They became sick of living in decline and constantly
> failing at different fitness and diet routines, knowing it
> was only going to get worse if they didn't change course.

I arm them with knowledge—weekly workout plans, *proper* execution of biomechanics (exercise form) during workout sessions, cardiovascular bouts with targeted heart rate zones, and nutritional profiles and plans, i.e., macros, micros, and supplements. All this is done by activating The FITNESS QUADRANT and then acclimating them to my trademarked system, called Modified Interval Training (MIT). This is where the anabolic pump gets primed and growth gets accessed by pulling in different scientific triggers that are leveraged through specific patterns and intervals. My clients are revered in the gym by other members, who literally stop and watch them as they perform detailed targeted movements and targeted patterns that take advantage of internal systems like adenosine triphosphate and phosphocreatine (ATP-PC) timing, contractile velocity applications, biomechanically correct structured movements, specific timing intervals, and adequate load (intensity) volume and frequency. There is so much involved in the MIT training system, it could be a book all on its own.

I have gratefully written thousands of different workouts, from post-surgical rehab modalities to high-level sport-specific performance modalities for pro athletes. I've had the pleasure of training hundreds of eager people—individuals ranging from doctors to bodybuilders, middle-aged moms and dads, grandparents, siblings, and also in groups (national teams) ranging from young high school, collegiate, and pro athletes to men and women in their 70s and 80s. No matter who is working out, it all comes down to understanding how to design training and nutritional platforms that are targeted at the intended outcome of that certain individual. So many things matter.

A wide-ranging set of skills is a requirement for this, and it has to be based on sound scientific principles and adequate experience. For example, someone who is 63 years old, sedentary, has bad knees and shoulder mobility issues, is obese, perhaps is completely intimidated at the thought of fitness, and is looking to lose 60 pounds of body fat requires different training protocols and timelines than an athlete who is looking to increase their speed, power, and agility as they chase and compete for a big, fat multimillion-dollar contract. One of the most important parts of what drives *all* their successes is their commitment to the correct process. It's not about just showing up to the gym. That's the easy part. It's about knowing the correct movements, timing, and routines to implement. They have to commit to learning the program in order to get better, or it will be a loss for everyone involved.

TESTIMONIALS

"In all my years of fitness and working with personal trainers (and getting injured), I have never been able to work out this little and get such dramatic results. Wow. I am now in control of my health." —

Sharry, 66 "In my twenty years as a clinical physical therapist, I've evaluated and rehabilitated thousands of bodies—from injured athletes to aging adults just trying to stay mobile. I've seen every fitness trend and gimmick come and go. But what Ward has created with The FITNESS QUADRANT and MIT method is, hands down, the most intelligent, results-driven, and biomechanically sound system I've ever encountered.

"This program isn't just for one age group—it gets modified for every level. Whether you're 45 or 75, the way Timothy integrates strength, mobility, cardiovascular conditioning, and recovery is on a level I've never seen. His attention to movement patterns, joint mechanics, and muscle sequencing is masterful. The precision of his biomechanics coaching alone is worth its weight in gold.

"Ward's FITNESS QUADRANT and his MIT method is the future of sustainable, science-based fitness. It's not just effective—it's exceptional." —Dan Fleury, MPT, clinical physical therapist with over twenty years in rehabilitation and human performance

"As doctors, we are expected to help people in any way we can, even outside of our trained medical field. I have never been more stunned than by the science and technical systems in The FITNESS QUADRANT and MIT method. Not only has it changed my body and health status, but it's beyond my medical pedigree." —Dr. "T" Shaib, 38

"The learning curve of MIT system is relatively short but, amazingly, will last a lifetime. Losing fat and gaining muscle, mobility, and energy is not only achievable but sustainable." —John S., 71

"Finding out that I have been doing fitness wrong my whole life is sort of enraging but also very liberating at the same time. I'm 60 pounds down! The FITNESS QUADRANT is genius." —Dr. Betty, PhD, 70

"I wish everybody who has a gym membership or who wants to finally get in shape would shut up and listen! You may think you know how to work out and eat properly, but guess what, you don't. After twenty-two years of working out incorrectly, this has been a game changer. I'm in better shape now than in my 30s." —Jay H., 56

"I have worked out my entire adult life (twenty-six years), and I have also been a certified fitness instructor, teaching classes and individuals for years. Wow, did I ever 'not know what I didn't know.' I started training with Tim and got introduced to The FITNESS QUADRANT and the MIT training method. With only two workouts per week (sometimes three), and with just 45-minute workouts, I have lost a lot of stubborn fat and have gained about 5 pounds of muscle and have had huge increases in my strength in only six months. And *no injuries*! This is profound fitness science all connected." —Lois S., 54

ASK YOURSELF SOME QUESTIONS:

If you had to define your fitness routine and your fitness level, what would it be?

Would you say your fitness routine is bad? Horrible? Okay? Pretty good? Kind of good? Great? Why?

When you walk into a gym, do you really know how to start and end a proper workout? Do you know how to perform a proper squat? Lat pulldown? Curl? Rowing motion? Do you know how many reps to do and why?

Have you ever wondered why you aren't in better shape? Or are you happy with how you look and feel?

Do you ever wonder if what you're doing for fitness is really working for you? Or do you just go along without any analysis?

Do you ever worry about the future you and your health level?

What is your plan for combating the aging process and increasing your quality of life, not just your longevity?

CHAPTER 4

THE CURRENT STATE OF HEALTH IN SOCIETY

It's happening to all of us. Every day, every minute, every second. We're all aging. We can't stop it. But we can influence it, slow it down. However, only a few of us have the knowledge to influence it. Most people will not prioritize learning the knowledge because it's very hard to find the right information. A small percentage of us have had the right channels to access proper exercise protocols and longevity sciences and then have had a large enough sample size of training people to assess the transformations.

A large portion of living strong and healthy is about what to avoid. Much of our world is toxic, as I continue to emphasize. It's designed to make profits—trillions—at the expense of your health. The cheap, toxic seed oils in 90% of your food, manufactured processed foods, toxic chemicals, fake sugar, and trans fats in our food supply are controlled by massive global companies whose sole mission is to make billions every year by selling cheap, addictive food. Add into this toxic, cancer-causing cookware, PBAs in plastics, and chemicals in the receipts at every checkout counter. These things, and virtually everything else we touch, have been linked to chemicals that degrade our bodies and literally kill us slowly. The more you know about it, the more you can avoid these toxic pieces that are all around us.

Living strong and healthy requires knowledge and experience. Knowing how to combine proper fitness protocols, nutritional habits, and, if needed, regenerative medicines, will make you literally—in comparison to everyone else on the planet—become a superhuman. Very fit, healthy, and strong.

Let's go on a journey. I hope I captivate your imagination so that it becomes your reality. This is my shining light. I am passing it on to you so you can pass the light on to your loved ones. Let's soar. Isn't it time for you to bite the bullet and get moving toward strong and healthy instead of weakness and decay? Think about that—living strong instead of weak. Decay or growth? You choose. Maybe it's not time for you to bite the bullet. Maybe you have to wait until you have a heart attack or until you can barely walk up the stairs because your knees are so sore or you're out of breath or until one of your loved ones suffers something traumatic that is directly related to health.

AMERICA IS RAPIDLY GROWING SICKER AND WEAKER

Here are three charts that tell the story:

Nationwide obesity rates have more than tripled since the 1960s.

Age-adjusted nationwide obesity and severe obesity rates according to National Health and Nutrition Examination Surveys

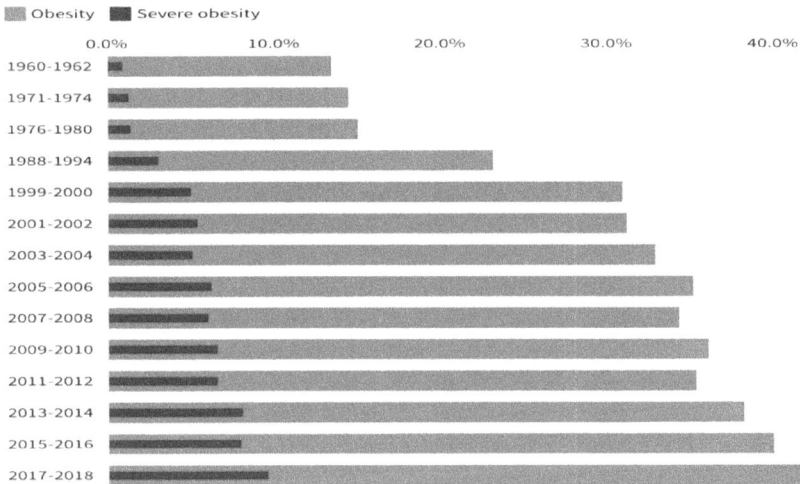

Obesity ■ Severe obesity

	0.0%	10.0%	20.0%	30.0%	40.0%
1960-1962					
1971-1974					
1976-1980					
1988-1994					
1999-2000					
2001-2002					
2003-2004					
2005-2006					
2007-2008					
2009-2010					
2011-2012					
2013-2014					
2015-2016					
2017-2018					

This accounts for the population between the ages of 20-74. The obesity category already includes severe obesity.

Source: Centers for Disease Control and Prevention, National Center for Health Statistics

USA FACTS

47

US FAST FOOD INDUSTRY MARKET SIZE OVER TIME

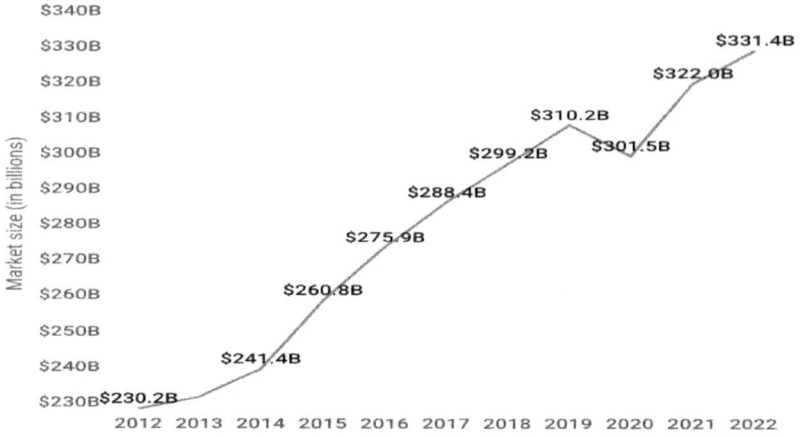

US PHARMACEUTICAL INDUSTRY REVENUE OVER TIME

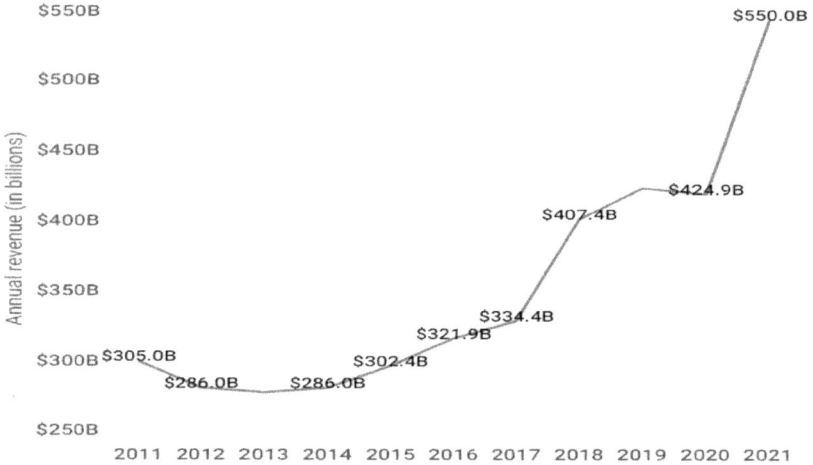

Notice how similar the growth of fast food and Big Pharma drug sales are.

1985: LEGALIZED DRUG ADVERTISING DIRECT TO CONSUMERS

The 1980s marked a historic period for Big Pharma and its extremely powerful lobby. America was about to become overmedicated—legally. Few people know that this was when the government made it legal for drug companies to advertise directly to consumers on radio and television. As a result, the corruption machine started to wind up, and your local doctors started making robust income from kickbacks for writing prescriptions from the big drug companies. America is one out of only three countries in the world that allow this. Direct-to-consumer (DTC) pharmaceutical advertising underwent a significant transformation in the United States starting in the 1980s. This shift allowed drug companies to advertise directly to consumers, several regulatory shifts in the 1980s by the FDA played a critical role in this practice.

Initially, DTC pharmaceutical advertising was sparse because of FDA regulations requiring detailed disclosure of side effects and risks, making it impractical for television and radio. However, in 1985, the FDA began clarifying rules for DTC ads, permitting them provided they met certain new disclosure standards that were much looser. This led to the gradual rise in such advertisements in print and broadcast media. Another significant shift occurred in the late 1990s when the FDA relaxed some of the guidelines further, particularly for television ads, requiring only a "major statement" of risks instead of a full list, significantly boosting the prevalence of such ads.

The practice of DTC pharmaceutical advertising remains controversial, with critics pointing to its role in overmedication and its influence on consumer demand for specific branded drugs, often at higher costs than their generic counterparts.

The US pharmaceutical industry is a controversial topic, but there is no denying that it is a huge part of the economy and has produced some life-saving drugs. It has also brought many new troubles and problems for society. As their revenue has increased, so too has the massive spike in new "ailments" that require new drugs for millions of people who think they are all magic pills that bring health benefits. Nothing could be more troubling than to see this mass psychosis. If anything, we have formed and developed a new mass addiction to pharmaceuticals. These drugs, marketed under false pretenses, have given birth to legalized addiction and a spike in depression in society, as well as a fast track to decay—*living weak and sick*. Once again, we see big profits, big banks, rich politicians—all making money off the backs of you, your family and children, and your good friends and neighbors. Disgusting.

Here are a few noteworthy statistics about pharmaceutical companies and consumers:

- The US pharmaceutical industry earned $550 billion in annual revenue in 2021.

- Americans spent $633.5 billion on medicine in 2022.

- The US is projected to spend $605–$635 billion on medicine in 2025.

- The US's pharmaceutical market accounts for 43.7% of the global pharmaceutical market in 2023.

So, if drugs are so helpful, why are people becoming sicker and unhealthier as reflected in the obesity growth curve that mirrors exactly the pharma sales growth curve? Why is that?

CHILDREN AND THE SEVENTY-TWO JABS: THE EXPLOSION OF AUTISM

Before we get into the increase in vaccination schedules below, I want to address the importance of taking care of our young ones in our country. It saddens me to my core to see the young children in our society sucking down toxic-laden energy drinks, sodas, fast foods, sugar-laced snacks, fake potato chips, French fries, candy, and "power bars." For the love of God, please stop your kids from eating like this. It is sending them off a cliff by the time they are in their 30s and 40s with all sorts of health problems. These gigantic global companies that make and distribute and market this poison disgust me. They know exactly what they are pushing. They only care about profits. Protect your kids and teach them, please. They are the future.

Increase in vaccination schedules:

- **1960s:** Children typically received vaccines for five diseases: diphtheria, tetanus, pertussis (DTP), polio, and smallpox.

- **2020s:** Children now receive vaccines for over sixteen diseases, including measles, mumps, rubella (MMR), hepatitis B, rotavirus, chickenpox, pneumococcal disease, and HPV.

According to the Centers for Disease Control and Prevention (CDC), the number of recommended doses increased from five in 1960 to over seventy-two by 2023, including boosters. The CDC attributes this expansion to advancements in medical science, targeting diseases with significant morbidity and mortality. Um, right.

Increase in autism rates:

- **1960s:** Estimated prevalence of autism was 1 in 2,500 children.

- **2023:** The CDC reports a prevalence of 1 in 36 children, with diagnoses being more common in boys.

If all these prescription drugs that are being pushed by doctors are so helpful and so good, then why are these autism numbers an absolute disaster? You know why. These are weapons of mass destruction. This disgusts me.

NOT ENOUGH FOR YOU? HOW ABOUT HEPATITIS B VAX, SHALL WE?

Every year in the United States, approximately 3.6 million babies are born. Within hours of life, nearly 3 million of them receive the Hepatitis B vaccine. Yet only about 18,000 of these infants are actually born to mothers carrying Hepatitis B—the only group truly at risk of transmission at birth.

This means that 99.6% of newborns are given a vaccine they *do not need*. At nearly $90 per injection, this practice generates *hundreds of millions of dollars* in revenue for pharmaceutical companies.

This is not about protecting newborns—it is about creating lifelong customers from the very first day outside the womb.

What makes this even more disturbing is the content of the shot itself. The Hepatitis B vaccine contains 250 micrograms of aluminum, a well-documented neurotoxin. To put this into perspective, that is far more than a fragile, hours-old infant's body can safely process. Research has linked aluminum exposure to neurological damage, autoimmune disorders, developmental delays, and even Alzheimer's disease later in life.

Yet this injection is administered to perfectly healthy babies who face virtually no risk of contracting Hepatitis B, all to pad profit margins. The risks are real. The benefits, for most infants, are nearly nonexistent. The math is simple—our children are being treated as currency.

If this reality makes your stomach turn, you are not alone. Parents deserve facts, not marketing slogans disguised as medical truth. Oh, the conflicts of interest that most doctors never reveal.

Nearly half of all deaths in 2021 were caused by heart disease, cancer, and COVID-19.

Top 10 leading causes of death in the US, 2021

Underlying cause of death	Total deaths
Heart Disease	695,547
Cancer	605,213
COVID-19	416,893
Accidents (unintentional injuries)	224,935
Stroke	162,890
Chronic lower respiratory diseases	142,342
Alzheimer's disease	119,399
Diabetes	103,294
Chronic liver disease and cirrhosis	56,585
Kidney disease	54,358

Kidney disease here refers to nephritis, nephrotic syndrome and nephrosis. Stroke refers to all cerebrovascular diseases.

Source: Centers for Disease Control and Prevention

USA**FACTS**

ANNUAL SLIP AND FALLS

Do you think strength, mobility, and balance are *not* an issue as we age? Look at these statistics from the CDC:

CDC Facts About Older Adult Falls

- About 36 million falls are reported among older adults each year—resulting in more than 32,000 deaths.

- Each year, about 3 million older adults are treated in emergency departments for a fall injury.

- One out of every five falls causes an injury, such as broken bones or a head injury.

- Each year, at least 300,000 older people are hospitalized for hip fractures.

- More than 95% of hip fractures are caused by falling—usually by falling sideways.

- Women fall more often than men and account for three quarters of all hip fractures.

- Slip and fall: Broken hip problems from slip and falls in age 55 and older.

Falls are a leading cause of injury among older adults, and broken hips are a common and serious consequence of these falls. According to the CDC, falls are the leading cause of injury-related death among adults aged 65 and older. In the US, falls are also the leading cause of nonfatal injuries among older adults, with more than 2.8 million older adults being treated in emergency departments for fall injuries each year.

The risk of falls and broken hips increases with age. The CDC reports that adults aged 55 and older are at higher risk for falls and fall-related injuries. Among older adults, about 1 in 4 will fall each year and 1 in 5 falls results in a serious injury, such as a broken bone or head injury.

Broken hips are particularly serious for older adults. The CDC estimates that about 300,000 older adults are hospitalized for hip fractures each year in the United States. Among older adults who fracture their hips, 20%–30% will die within a year, and 25%–50% will require long-term care.

In summary, falls are a major problem among older adults, particularly those aged 55 and older. The risk of falls and fall-related injuries, such as broken hips, increases with age. The CDC estimates that falls are the leading cause of injury-related death among adults aged 65 and older and the leading cause of nonfatal injuries among older adults. Broken hips, in particular, are a serious consequence of falls among older adults, with about 300,000 older adults hospitalized for hip fractures each year in the United States.

SKINNY JIMMY – PART 1

There I was, training a new client who was so typical. Amanda, a CPA, was 57 years old and 55 pounds overweight. She had a bad right knee, a very tight left hip, and a lower back that was so unstable it would be randomly thrown out of whack four times a year at the slightest movement and then go on to become debilitating for weeks at a time. You know, the back thing—can't put your socks or shoes on without a struggle because it is flared up and painful. Can't get out of a chair, a car, or bed in the morning effortlessly and easily. You have to go slow because your back is so tight and you might tweak it if you go too fast and risk having it seize up again. Yeah, the back thing.

While explaining various exercise movements to Amanda, I saw this guy out of the corner of my eye eavesdropping with more intensity than the other members who were on the gym floor trying to exercise. And he wasn't hiding it either! Amanda and I were covering very important topics on biomechanics, the technical term for exercise form. Improper biomechanics is how a vast majority of people hurt their lower backs, shoulders, and knees. Out of nowhere, this guy watching and listening to us, which happens to be Skinny Jimmy, says, "That's the reason my back and shoulders always hurt!"

We all kind of chuckled at him, and I kindly said, "Yes, you're right, because I've watched some of the exercises you're doing, and unfortunately, your form is incorrect. That's why you're injured. Biomechanics is so important. They actually dictate whether or not your resistance training is legitimate and helpful. It's that simple."

I could also tell by how severely skinny he was that he also had a major problem with his nutrition. At 6'1", he was only 149 pounds. I wanted to go into the topic, but it was not my place to do so at the time. Thankfully, I made a new friend that day, and unbeknownst to me, it was the beginning of a long trainer-client relationship that would become one of the most transformative success stories I've seen in thirty-five years.

Unfortunately, 95% of gym members do not know how to execute even basic exercises or even engage a workout properly, and they end up completely missing out on the most important benefits of working out—that's millions of gym-goers every day in the world. Sad but true. With a little education and some guidance, this could dramatically change.

But back to Amanda and the biomechanics instruction. This is an area where I always take a deeper dive into the vital topic with everyone I work with, no exceptions. This education process is a requirement of mine. They must go through it or I decline to take them on. This involves learning to understand things like the frontal plane, sagittal plane, transverse plane, rotational planes, pelvic girdle tilt, femoral head position during hip extension movements, synovial joint mechanics, Golgi tendon organs and the central nervous system (CNS), eccentric versus concentric contractions, contractile velocity, motor unit recruitment patterns, intensity levels, synchronous and asynchronous firing patterns, just to name a few points. It has become my trademark of how I onboard every client, giving them an inside view of what high-quality resistance training *actually is*. I teach them how joints are not only protected through this process but also how they strengthen and gain increased integrity and range of motion over time. And how muscles fire properly through a voluntary contractile recruitment process that triggers a much larger percentage of contractile proteins called actin and myosin to fire, and how this process unleashes a tsunami of hormonal rivers through the bloodstream. This includes interleukin 10 (IL-10)—a major growth hormone that signals the body to turn on anabolic machinery and simultaneously turn off the inflammation hormone interleukin 6 (IL-6), which is a decay (catabolic) hormone. I also teach them how bones gain more density and integrity when the connective tissue is pulled on by muscle, in turn pulling on the bones and triggering an adaptive response signaling the bones to get thicker and stronger.

As I recall, I had seen Skinny Jimmy in the gym for months at that point. It seemed like every time I was training myself or with clients, he was always there, frantically moving throughout the gym for hours. Dedication was not his problem—a total lack of knowledge was. So I started to watch what he was doing a little more, and yes, he actually would get right next to me and my clients on a machine so he could observe us more closely. I mean, this guy went at it hard, and I admired his commitment and intensity. But wow. I looked at what he was doing, and then how he was doing it, and when I saw him doing movements that were destroying his lower back, knees, and shoulder joints, I couldn't keep my mouth shut any longer.

I rarely give advice in the gym. I stay in my lane even though I am bursting at the seams to help people. So I asked the fitness gods in my mind, "Can I please say something to this man so I can help him *not* wreck his body anymore?" And then I waited for my moment—all in the name of helping him, by the way.

Alright, he was doing upright rows and wincing. He was completely destroying his rotator cuffs with one of the worst exercises you could ever do with weights. I couldn't take it anymore. I had to say something… But wait a minute! Here he was, walking over to me like a person possessed! He said, "You got a second?"

I replied, "I sure do. What's up?"

Jimmy said, "I'd like to hire you. How do you work with people?"

SECTION 1 TAKEAWAYS

- Know the truth about what causes accelerated aging and how to reverse it.

- By choice or by consequence, fitness and health will become a major priority in your wellness story at some point.

- There is an appropriate entry point for everyone in a weekly fitness and wellness routine.

- Prioritize your well-being and your muscle-gaining plan.

- Learn the right way to make yourself stronger and healthier.

- There are no get-fit-quick products. They are all scams. Legitimate exercise science practices, deep experience, and expert coaching lead the way.

- Commit to just three hours per week of a proper fitness routine and you'll flourish.

SECTION 2
YOUR TOXIC WORLD

The origins of weapons of mass destruction to our health are toxic soils and crops, toxic processed food, and Big Pharma. The roots and precursors that affect our lives so severely include:

- Unbalanced soils, lab-altered seeds, chemical crops

- Mass-produced "factory food" and toxic products

- Over-prescribed and unnecessary pharmaceuticals

A devastating one-two-three punch to all of us. It all starts with nutrient-deficient crops, caused by the chemical fertilizers, unbalanced agricultural soils, genetically altered seeds, and toxic soil management practices, along with chemical spray applications to manage infestation. This is Big Ag and big business. We get sick from a toxic food supply, then we run to our doctors for loads of prescription meds that are supposed to fix the problem but only lead to more prescriptions. Don't even get me started on the new rage of GLP-1 semaglutide "weight-loss drugs" like Wegovy, Ozempic, Rybelsus... Talk about losing muscle mass and bone density at the speed of light. Whoa. There are now thousands of lawsuits against these weight-loss drug makers. Nah, nothing wrong here. The new forever drugs that deteriorate your body from the inside out. This is pure insanity. This is called sickness management, and it is *not* a solution. It's a gigantic problem for society—adding even more to the $4.3 trillion annually, in fact. Never ever forget, depression is a business. Hypertension is a business. Diabetes is a business. Cancer is a business. And it is big, big business. *None* of these businesses profit or even exist if you're healthy or cured.

The real solution starts before the food even hits your plate—by fixing the soil it's grown in by eliminating the chemical inputs while simultaneously stopping the herbicides and pesticides spraying.

Nutrient-rich food comes from healthy, toxin-free soil. That's how you avoid eating produce that's quietly breaking you down instead of building you up. Combine that with the proper fitness and health ecosystem, i.e., The FITNESS QUADRANT, and you've got a formula to become strong, energized, and damn near unstoppable.

Do you want to be truly healthy? This is one of the first things you need to learn about and understand more clearly if you want to live in growth mode, not decay mode. There is so much to write about that it cannot possibly fit into one book, let alone a section in this book. We'll cover some of it and shed some light on the topic so you can peek behind the curtain a little in the next section. I am really hoping it hits home and opens your eyes. Even better, I hope you take action and make changes in your life.

Remember one of the major takeaways of this book: even the best fitness routines in the world are virtually destroyed by toxic nutrition. Beware of the fake labels that act like the companies are your friend. The poisonous food industry is at its worst when they disguise their brands as "Organic" and "Natural" and "Fresh." Labeling laws need to be completely overhauled in the US. What looks healthy and wholesome is usually laced with toxic fake sugars, chemical food extenders, color additives (like BP-40), trans fats, and rancid, inflammatory seed oils. Want an example? How about Kind bars. When you look at the ingredients, you'll see they're not so "kind."

Learning how to spot this trash and what to avoid is the first step to growing strong.

LEARN A LESSON FROM THE AMISH PLEASE

Americans are growing sicker than ever. There are many smaller countries and cultures that are much healthier as a whole than the big Ole USA. Here is a brief example and look at the lifestyle of the Amish who have impressive health and longevity statistics when compared to the rest of the US population:

Americans VS. Amish: A Remarkable Health Contrast

The Amish community has just a 4% obesity rate—that's nine times lower than the average American.

They don't count calories.

They don't touch mass produced foods.

They don't obsess or participate in "fad" trendy health routines.

They don't take pharmaceuticals.

Yet they are leaner, stronger, and living longer than 96% of America.

So, what's their secret?

- Their food isn't poisoned. They eat real food, unprocessed and free from toxins, rich in whole animal proteins
- No refined sugar. No seed oils—butter, tallow, and olive oil instead.
- They move daily with farming, manual labor, and craftsmanship as their exercise.
- They have 63% lower muscle loss and 42% better cognitive function than Americans.
- An average Amish person walks three to four times more than the average American person.
- They live free from toxic chemicals, zero vaccines.
- Their sense of purpose, community, and connection keeps them young.

Meanwhile…

Most of us in America are drowning in ultra-processed food, addiction to pharmaceuticals, blue light, hidden toxins, and all the toxic designer personal care products under the sun while wondering why disease and fatigue have become the "new normal."

The Amish don't *chase* health. Their lifestyle simply creates it.

CHAPTER 1

THE FOUR
DARK HORSEMEN

The four dark horsemen are slowly killing America while making billions for themselves and the big firms on Wall Street, Big Pharma, and the medical industry. These industries are some of the biggest donors to politicians through big-time lobbyists. Nothing suspicious here though.

Of the food sold in grocery stores today, 95% *did not exist* one hundred years ago. Neither did 95% of the chronic diseases. Funny how that works, isn't it?

1. SEED OILS

Widely used in the American diet, seed oils have raised concerns due to their destructive health impacts, particularly their links to inflammation and chronic diseases. These oils, derived from seeds such as soybeans, corn, sunflower, and cottonseed, became a dietary staple in the twentieth century as by-products of industrial processes. Their affordability and long shelf life made them ideal for mass food production, but they are nutritionally and chemically problematic. Chemical solvents like hexane are often used in seed oil production, and synthetic antioxidants are added to prolong shelf life. These additives carry potential risks, including endocrine disruption and carcinogenic effects. Seed oils emerged as industrial by-products, with the earliest uses in non-food industries like soap and engine/machinery lubricant production. Over time, marketing positioned them as healthier alternatives to saturated fats. From the 1970s to the early 2000s, seed oil consumption in the US skyrocketed, with soybean oil intake increasing sixfold, now accounting for a significant portion of caloric intake.

In the realm of nutrition, the perilous path of modern dietary habits has led us into a realm fraught with dangers—the unchecked consumption of seed oils. Once heralded as a healthier alternative than butter and tallow, these oils have now come under scrutiny for their toxicity and adverse health effects. I will delve into the intricacies of this issue, uncovering a web of scientific evidence, including studies from researchers such as Paul Saladino, MD, that shed light on the dangers of seed oils. I will also explore the alarming prevalence of these oils in processed foods and their contribution to the growing health crisis.

Unraveling the Seed Oil Quandary

Seed oils, often labeled as vegetable oils, are derived from the seeds of plants such as soybean, canola, corn, and sunflower. Despite their widespread use, mounting research suggests that these oils may pose significant health risks due to their high content of omega-6 fatty acids, which can lead to an imbalance in the omega-6 to omega-3 ratio. This imbalance has been directly linked to inflammation, oxidative stress, and an array of chronic health conditions, including heart disease, obesity, and metabolic syndrome.

Studies by esteemed researchers have contributed to this discourse. For instance, some have shown that excessive consumption of seed oils, particularly those rich in linoleic acid (a common omega-6 fatty acid), may promote inflammation and negatively impact arterial function. These findings underscore the need for a critical reevaluation of the role of seed oils in our diets.

A Stealthy Culprit in Processed Foods

The pervasive presence of seed oils in processed foods is cause for heightened concern. These oils have infiltrated a vast array of products, including baked goods, condiments, and snack foods, pervading our diets in ways we may not even realize. Restaurants, too, often employ seed oils for cooking and frying due to their affordability and stability under high heat.

The ubiquity of seed oils in processed foods is alarming, given their potential to contribute to health problems. By carefully scrutinizing ingredient labels and understanding the aliases of these oils (such as soybean oil or corn oil), individuals can make more informed choices about the foods they consume, thereby minimizing their exposure to these potentially harmful substances.

The Top Eight Seed Oils to Avoid at All Costs

Several seed oils dominate the market and make their way into countless products. The top eight seed oils by annual dollar sales and volume in tonnage are:

1. Soybean oil
2. Canola oil
3. Palm oil
4. Corn oil
5. Sunflower oil
6. Cottonseed oil
7. Safflower oil
8. Rapeseed oil (term used for canola oil)

These oils collectively contribute to a massive industry, but their widespread use comes at a steep cost to public health. Again, the unaware, unknowing public are the ones who suffer the greatest consequences.

The toxic undercurrent of seed oils in our diets is a pressing concern that demands our attention. The mounting evidence of their potential harm, coupled with their omnipresence in processed foods, calls for a reevaluation of dietary habits. By being mindful of ingredient labels, choosing cooking oils with a balanced omega-6 to omega-3 ratio, and emphasizing whole, minimally processed foods, individuals can take proactive steps to minimize their exposure to seed oils and safeguard their health.

As the scientific community continues to uncover the intricacies of seed oils and their impact on health, it is incumbent upon us to navigate this complex terrain with knowledge and discernment. The journey toward optimal health requires a commitment to informed choices and a proactive approach to reshaping our diets. In doing so, we will pave the way for a future characterized by vitality and well-being, free from the potential hazards that lurk within our food supply.

The Top Five Cancer-Causing Toxic Seed Oils Found in Grocery Stores

1. **Canola Oil:** Canola oil, also known as rapeseed oil, has been shown to contain high levels of erucic acid, a toxic compound that has been linked to heart damage and cancer. Studies have also found that canola oil can promote the growth of tumors and inhibit the growth of healthy cells.

2. **Cottonseed Oil:** Cottonseed oil has been found to contain high levels of gossypol, a toxic compound that can cause cancer. Studies have also found that cottonseed oil can promote the growth of tumors and inhibit the growth of healthy cells.

3. **Soybean Oil:** Soybean oil has been found to contain high levels of phytoestrogens, compounds that can mimic the effects of estrogen in the body. This can lead to an increased risk of cancer, particularly in women.

4. **Sunflower Oil:** Sunflower oil has been found to contain high levels of omega-6 fatty acids, which can promote inflammation in the body. This can lead to an increased risk of cancer, as well as other chronic health conditions.

5. **Corn Oil:** Corn oil has been found to contain high levels of omega-6 fatty acids, which can promote inflammation in the body. This can lead to an increased risk of cancer, as well as other chronic health conditions.

Consuming seed oils can cause the following health impacts:

1. **Inflammation:** Seed oils are rich in omega-6 fatty acids, which, in excess, contribute to an imbalanced omega-6 to omega-3 ratio. While both are essential fats, excessive omega-6 promotes the production of pro-inflammatory molecules, exacerbating chronic inflammation linked to conditions like heart disease, arthritis, and metabolic disorders.

2. **Oxidative Stress:** These oils are highly prone to oxidation due to their polyunsaturated fat content. When exposed to heat and light during cooking, they generate harmful by-products such as free radicals and lipid peroxides, which damage cells and DNA, increasing the risk of chronic diseases.

3. **Gut Health:** Seed oils may disrupt the gut microbiome, weakening gut lining integrity and contributing to inflammation and gastrointestinal disorders.

What are the good oils?

If you want to thrive in a growth mode—anabolic mode—you must eliminate seed oils as you now know, or at the very least, minimize seed oil intake by avoiding all processed foods and favoring alternatives like high quality olive oil, avocado oil, beef tallow, and pure butter. These are the good ones that the US government officials lied to the public about for decades as they gave favor to the massive multi-billion dollar processed food giants' buddies that in turn help fund their campaigns. They went on an intentional deceptive smear campaign against butter, egg yolks, and saturated fats as dangerous foods that cause heart attacks and then praised alternatives like Crisco shortening, margarine, and vegetable and canola oil that ultimately translated into billions of dollars of corporate profits for the fake chemical stuff. Disgusting.

These natural options—or what I like to call God's food—offer much healthier fat profiles and are less prone to oxidation. Prioritizing a balanced intake of omega-3-rich foods like fish and flaxseeds can also help correct the omega-6 to omega-3 imbalance, promoting overall health.

2. FAKE SUGAR (A.K.A. ARTIFICIAL SWEETENERS)

Often marketed as "natural sweetener" or "natural flavoring," these fake sugars have become pervasive in the American diet, widely used as substitutes for sugar in various products to lower calorie content. Despite their popularity, research suggests they may cause a variety of health issues, including inflammation, insulin dysregulation, diabetes, metabolic damage, and addiction to sweet tastes.

Consuming artificial sweeteners can cause the following health impacts:

1. **Inflammation and Gut Health:** Artificial sweeteners like sucralose and saccharin have been linked to changes in gut microbiota and gastrointestinal inflammation. Dysbiosis caused by these sweeteners may contribute to conditions such as inflammatory bowel disease (IBD) and metabolic disorders.

2. **Insulin and Metabolism:** Studies indicate artificial sweeteners can impair glucose metabolism and insulin sensitivity, leading to an increased risk of type 2 diabetes. High consumers of sweeteners, particularly aspartame and sucralose, have been found to face significantly higher risks of developing diabetes.

3. **Obesity and Addiction:** Artificial sweeteners, being much sweeter than sugar, may alter taste preferences, causing a massive increase and cravings for highly sweetened foods. Ironically, they are associated with weight gain rather than weight loss, as they are clearly shown to disrupt appetite regulation. This is a huge problem that causes an avalanche of larger problems.

Artificial sweeteners were first introduced in the late nineteenth century, with saccharin being the earliest example. Their usage surged in the mid-twentieth century as the food industry sought cost-effective sugar substitutes. Over the past fifty years, the consumption of these sweeteners has grown significantly, and they are now estimated to be present in over 23,000 products, including beverages, processed foods, and even medications.

These fake sugars are cheap to produce and up to 20,000 times sweeter than sugar, making them highly cost-effective for manufacturers. This economic advantage has contributed to their widespread adoption. Between 1999 and 2012, consumption of these sweeteners increased by 200% in children and 54% in adults, highlighting their growing presence in the food supply.

While precise numbers vary, their market presence aligns with the rise in obesity and metabolic syndromes in developed nations. Here are two graphs spotlighting trends:

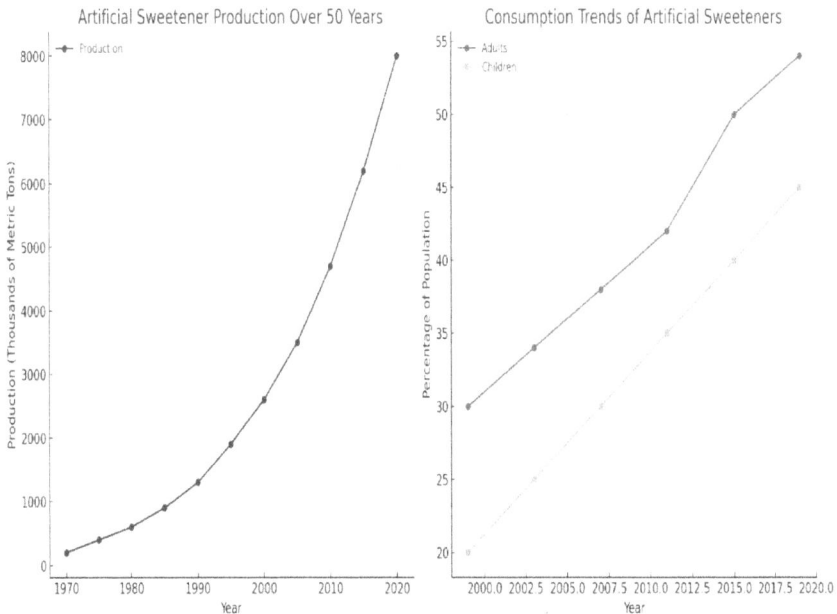

1. **Production Over Time:** The first graph shows the dramatic increase in artificial sweetener production over the past fifty years, reflecting their integration into the global food system. Production has risen from 200,000 metric tons in 1970 to approximately 8 million metric tons by 2020.

2. **Consumption Trends in the US:** The second graph highlights the growing prevalence of artificial sweetener use among adults and children. Consumption rates have increased steadily, with 54% of adults and 45% of children consuming these sweeteners by 2019.

3. TRANS FATS

Perhaps one of the greatest health scams in history. Chemically manufactured trans fats have their origins in the early twentieth century, specifically in 1901, when German chemist Wilhelm Normann developed a process to hydrogenate liquid oils, transforming them into solid or semi-solid fats. This process, patented in 1902, involved bubbling hydrogen gas through vegetable or fish oils to create more stable and solid fats.

Normann's invention led to the production of the first hydrogenated shortening, Crisco, by Procter & Gamble in 1911. Crisco, made from partially hydrogenated cottonseed oil, was marketed as a cheaper and more durable alternative to butter and lard. The product gained popularity due to its longer shelf life and versatility in cooking and baking.

By the mid-twentieth century, trans fats had become a staple in many food products, including margarine, shortening, baked goods, and fried foods. Here is a brief overview of their growth in the human diet:

- **Pre-1970s:** Trans fats were increasingly used in food products as a substitute for saturated fats, which were perceived as unhealthy. This led to a significant rise in trans-fat consumption.

- **1970s–1980s:** Preliminary studies began to suggest that trans fats might be harmful, but they were still widely used. Reviews by the FDA in 1976 and 1985 did not conclusively indicate harm, leading to continued high consumption.

- **1990s: Clinical and epidemiological studies** established clear evidence that industrially produced trans fats were linked to heart disease. This led to a decline in their use, but they remained prevalent in many food products.

- **2006 and Beyond:** The FDA mandated that food labels list trans-fat content, leading to a significant reduction in their consumption. By 2015, the FDA determined that partially hydrogenated oils, the primary source of artificial trans fats, were no longer "generally recognized as safe" and began phasing them out of food products. Today, the use of artificial trans fats is heavily restricted, and many countries have banned or limited their use.

Here are the top four harmful effects of trans fats:

1. Cardiovascular Disease

Trans fats increase levels of low-density lipoprotein (LDL) cholesterol and decrease levels of high-density lipoprotein (HDL) cholesterol. This imbalance can lead to the buildup of cholesterol in arteries, increasing the risk of heart disease and stroke.

2. Inflammation and Immune System Overactivity

Consuming trans fats promotes inflammation and overactivity of the immune system, which has been linked to various chronic conditions, including heart disease, stroke, diabetes, and other metabolic disorders.

3. Weight Gain and Insulin Resistance

Trans fats can contribute to weight gain and increase the risk of type 2 diabetes by promoting insulin resistance. Studies have shown that diets high in trans fats can lead to increased abdominal fat deposits and metabolic syndrome.

4. Cancer-Related Issues

Recent studies have linked trans-fat intake to an increased risk of certain cancers, including breast, prostate, and colorectal cancers. The exact mechanisms are not fully understood, but the association between trans-fat consumption and cancer risk is a significant concern.

In summary, the introduction of chemically manufactured trans fats revolutionized food production but has since been recognized as a major public health risk.

4. FOOD DYES

Artificial food dyes are widely used in processed foods to enhance visual appeal and product uniformity. All to sell more crap to you and your children. Yeah, that's right. It's psychological, we eat with our eyes.

However, these dyes pose significant health risks. The top three synthetic food dyes of concern include:

1. Red 40 (Allura Red AC)

- **Health Risks**: Linked to hyperactivity, behavioral issues in children, and allergic reactions. It may also contain impurities linked to cancer. Studies suggest it may cause potential DNA damage and oxidative stress in cells.

- **Usage**: Found in candy, baked goods, soft drinks, and more. It is the most commonly used food dye in the US.

2. Yellow 5 (Tartrazine)

- **Health Risks**: Causes hypersensitivity reactions, particularly in individuals with aspirin intolerance, and may contain carcinogenic contaminants. It's also linked to behavioral disturbances in children.

- **Usage**: Common in sodas, chips, and desserts.

3. Yellow 6 (Sunset Yellow)

- **Health Risks**: Associated with adrenal gland and kidney tumors in animal studies and contains contaminants like benzidine, a known carcinogen.
- **Usage**: Present in candies, beverages, and baked goods.

These dyes can disrupt hormones, cause inflammation, and negatively affect the gut microbiome, potentially leading to systemic issues like obesity and weakened immunity. Children are particularly vulnerable due to lower body weight and higher intake of processed foods relative to adults. Studies have also highlighted neurobehavioral impacts, especially in children with ADHD or autism.

Globally, the US leads in synthetic food dye usage, with estimates suggesting that children consume artificial dyes at levels far exceeding the amounts linked to behavioral effects in clinical trials. In contrast, the European Union mandates warning labels on products containing these dyes and some dyes are banned altogether.

There are alternatives! Natural dyes, such as those derived from turmeric, spinach, or beetroot, are less harmful and may even provide anti-inflammatory health benefits. The US is the only country that does not use these alternatives. Toxic artificial dyes are banned in other countries.

Wake up everybody, please!

CHAPTER 2

THE INVISIBLE ASSASSIN

Brought on by the three of the four dark horsemen, inflammation is the immune system's critical biological response to harmful stimuli such as pathogens, damaged cells, or irritants. However, chronic inflammation, often triggered by diet and lifestyle factors, can lead to numerous health issues, including cardiovascular diseases, diabetes, and autoimmune disorders. Chronic inflammation undermines the body's ability to heal and maintain homeostasis. Over time, it contributes to tissue damage, insulin resistance, and the onset of chronic diseases such as cancer, Alzheimer's, and metabolic syndrome.

CAUSES OF INFLAMMATION

1. **Seed Oils and Trans Fats:** Excess consumption of seed oils (rich in omega-6 fatty acids) and trans fats can trigger the production of pro-inflammatory chemicals in the body. This imbalance in fatty acid intake (high omega-6 versus low omega-3) promotes systemic inflammation, which is linked to heart disease, obesity, and arthritis.

2. **Artificial Sweeteners:** Artificial sweeteners like aspartame provoke an immune response. This reaction can exacerbate inflammation and other autoimmune symptoms.

3. **Refined Sugars:** Processed sugars stimulate the release of inflammatory cytokines, aggravating conditions such as

diabetes and heart disease. These sugars are found in numerous processed foods and beverages.

Inflammatory foods are those that can contribute to inflammation in the body, which can lead to chronic health conditions such as heart disease, diabetes, and cancer. Here are the top ten common inflammatory foods and drinks that can be found in grocery stores:

1. Processed meats, such as bacon, deli meat, and hot dogs – high in saturated fat and sodium

2. Refined carbohydrates, such as white bread, pasta, and pastries – can spike blood sugar levels

3. Fried foods, such as French fries, fried chicken, and doughnuts – high in unhealthy fats and trans fats

4. Sugar-sweetened beverages, such as soda, sports drinks, and energy drinks – high in added sugars

5. Artificial sweeteners, which are often found in diet and low-calorie foods – can disrupt the balance of gut bacteria

6. Margarine and shortening – high in trans fats

7. Processed snack foods, such as chips, crackers, and cookies – high in sodium and added sugars

8. Dairy products, particularly if you're lactose intolerant or suffer from dairy allergies

9. High-fat and grain-fed meats – may be high in saturated fats and pro-inflammatory omega-6 fatty acids

10. Alcohol in excessive amounts – can lead to inflammation in the liver and other organs

It's important to note that the above foods may not be inflammatory for everyone. It is best to consult with a doctor or a dietician if you have any concerns. Additionally, it's also important to eat a balanced diet that includes a variety of anti-inflammatory foods such as fruits, vegetables, whole grains, and lean proteins.

MITIGATION STRATEGIES

Dietary changes can significantly reduce inflammation. For instance:

- Increasing omega-3 fatty acid intake through fish, flaxseeds, and walnuts can help balance the pro-inflammatory effects of omega-6 fats.

- Avoiding foods with trans fats, artificial sweeteners, and excessive refined sugars can lower inflammation levels.

An anti-inflammatory diet focuses on whole, nutrient-dense foods that reduce inflammation while avoiding processed and pro-inflammatory foods.

Key foods to include:

1. **Fatty Fish:** Salmon, mackerel, and sardines are rich in omega-3 fatty acids, which counterbalance pro-inflammatory omega-6s.

2. **Fruits and Vegetables:** Berries, oranges, leafy greens, and cruciferous vegetables are high in antioxidants like vitamin C and polyphenols.

3. **Whole Grains:** Oats, quinoa, and brown rice provide fiber, which supports gut health and reduces systemic inflammation.

4. **Healthy Fats:** Avocados, nuts, seeds, and olive oil are anti-inflammatory fats.

5. **Spices:** Turmeric (curcumin) and ginger have natural anti-inflammatory properties.

Foods to avoid:

- Refined sugars and artificial sweeteners.

- Trans fats and excessive omega-6 oils (all seed oils, including soybean, corn, vegetable, canola).

- Processed foods with additives and preservatives.

Sample meals:

- **Breakfast:** Whole farm eggs & steak, ½ sourdough bagel with honey and almond butter, blueberries.
- **Lunch:** Grilled salmon over spinach, pears, walnuts, avocado, and olive oil dressing.
- **Dinner:** Red meat with roasted vegetables and grilled pineapple.
- **Snacks:** Fresh fruit, mixed nuts, Greek yogurt, beef jerky, protein bar.

SUPPLEMENTS FOR INFLAMMATION REDUCTION

While earth food is the cornerstone for a healthy diet, certain supplements can amplify anti-inflammatory effects, like:

1. **Omega-3 Fatty Acids:** High-quality fish oil supplements help reduce markers of inflammation like C-reactive protein (CRP).
2. **Curcumin:** Found in turmeric, curcumin reduces inflammation at the cellular level and is especially beneficial for joint health.
3. **Vitamin D:** Helps regulate immune responses and is linked to reduced inflammation in people with low levels.
4. **Probiotics:** Support gut health, which plays a crucial role in systemic inflammation.
5. **Magnesium:** Known to combat oxidative stress and inflammatory cytokines.

RESISTANCE TRAINING AND INFLAMMATION

Resistance training, such as weightlifting or bodyweight exercises, reduces inflammation through multiple mechanisms:

1. **Reduction in Pro-Inflammatory Cytokines:** Regular resistance training decreases levels of cytokines like TNF-alpha

and IL-6, which are linked to inflammation, while simultaneously increasing IL-10 (a major anti-inflammatory compound), which is referred to as "the cleaning crew" by exercise science researchers.

2. **Improved Insulin Sensitivity:** Exercise enhances the body's ability to regulate blood sugar, reducing inflammation associated with insulin resistance.

3. **Increased Muscle Mass:** Stronger muscles help combat age-related inflammation and metabolic disorders.

4. **Enhanced Antioxidant Defense:** Exercise boosts the production of endogenous antioxidants, reducing oxidative stress.

ANTI-INFLAMMATORY FOODS

These foods can help reduce inflammation in the body:

- Fruits and vegetables, especially those high in antioxidants like berries, cherries, and leafy greens

- Fatty fish such as salmon, mackerel, and sardines, which are high in omega-3 fatty acids

- Nuts and seeds, especially those high in anti-inflammatory compounds like almonds, walnuts, and flaxseeds

- Whole grains such as quinoa, oats, and brown rice

- Spices such as turmeric, ginger, and garlic, which contain compounds that have anti-inflammatory effects

It's important to note that a diet high in anti-inflammatory foods is generally considered to be healthier overall.

CHAPTER 3

THE FIFTH HORSEMAN

The public water supply in the US often contains several toxic chemicals, some of which have been linked to significant health risks, including cancer, endocrine disruption, and hormonal imbalances. Stop drinking and bathing in water from the public supply and get a high-quality filtration system.

KEY CHEMICALS AND HEALTH IMPACTS

Fluoride

Fluoride is added to public water systems to reduce tooth decay. It is a neurotoxin that disrupts and cause damage to the brain in humans. Its health benefits are and always have been fraudulent and totally without merit. Many studies that have actually been covered up have raised concerns about its effects on the endocrine system, particularly the thyroid. High fluoride intake has been associated with decreased levels of T3 and T4 hormones, critical for thyroid function, and potential interference with iodine metabolism. Some populations exposed to high fluoride levels have shown increased rates of skeletal fluorosis, endocrine abnormalities, and potential neurological impacts.

Atrazine

The chemical atrazine has been highlighted in public discussions, including by Robert F. Kennedy Jr., for its potential effects on both the environment and human health. Atrazine, a widely used herbicide, has been shown in research to disrupt endocrine systems. Studies, including those led by biologist Tyrone Hayes at UC Berkeley, indicate that atrazine can cause significant changes in amphibians. For example, male frogs exposed to atrazine at concentrations lower than the US Environmental Protection Agency's (EPA) safety thresholds exhibited feminization, chemical castration, and, in some cases, developed into fully functional females capable of producing viable eggs. These effects underscore concerns about atrazine's role as an endocrine disruptor.

Atrazine remains one of the most heavily used herbicides in the US and is present in approximately 63% of the country's water supply, although it is banned in many other countries. Its inclusion in drinking water has sparked debates about its potential impact on human health, particularly regarding hormonal disruptions and developmental effects. While extensive direct evidence of its effects on humans remains limited, some epidemiological studies have linked atrazine exposure to developmental and reproductive health issues, such as small-for-gestational-age babies in high-exposure areas.

PFAS (Per- and Polyfluoroalkyl Substances)

PFAS are known as "forever chemicals" due to their persistence in the environment and resistance to degradation. Commonly found in water supplies due to industrial discharge, these chemicals can disrupt hormonal systems, including thyroid function, and have been linked to cancer and developmental issues.

Other Endocrine Disruptors

Arsenic and various industrial by-products, including pesticides like glyphosate, have been detected in water supplies. Arsenic exposure, even at low levels, is linked to metabolic disorders, cardiovascular issues, and reproductive health problems.

Plastics and Microplastics

Microplastics in water can leach endocrine-disrupting chemicals, such as bisphenols and phthalates, which interfere with hormonal regulation and may contribute to developmental and cognitive deficits.

Again, many of these chemicals were introduced into water systems either intentionally, like fluoride for dental health, or unintentionally, through industrial waste. Over time, their potential health impacts have become evident, sparking debates about regulatory standards and safety.

A case in point—consequences now being realized, the EPA recently announced stricter guidelines for PFAS, limiting six specific compounds due to their widespread health effects.

Also, long-term studies have linked fluoride exposure to both skeletal and non-skeletal health risks, especially in populations with additional risk factors like iodine deficiency.

CHAPTER 4

COMMON TOXIC HOUSEHOLD PRODUCTS

You must become more aware of the hidden dangers in the world you live in. Here are just three examples out of hundreds of products you most likely have in your home right now and that, unfortunately, you and your family have unknowingly been using for years.

- plastic food containers and utensils

- paraffin candles

- sunscreens

Modern conveniences most often come with huge hidden health risks. Those three common items expose us to harmful chemicals with long-term health effects. Here's a closer look at their risks and the science behind them so you can be aware of these ticking time bombs.

PLASTIC FOOD CONTAINERS AND UTENSILS

Toxic Ingredients:

- **Bisphenol A (BPA) and Bisphenol S (BPS):** Common in hard plastics, these are endocrine disruptors.

- **Phthalates:** Found in flexible plastics, these chemicals increase malleability but can leach into food.

- **Polycyclic Aromatic Hydrocarbons (PAHs):** Released when plastic is exposed to heat or microwaved.

Harmful Effects:

- **Hormonal Disruption:** BPA and BPS mimic estrogen, potentially leading to fertility issues, early puberty, and hormone-related cancers (e.g., breast and prostate cancer).

- **Developmental Risks:** Prenatal exposure to phthalates has been linked to developmental delays in children.

- **Carcinogenic Potential:** PAHs released from heated plastics are known carcinogens.

- **Research Evidence:** A 2019 study in *Environmental Health Perspectives* found that BPA alternatives like BPS also disrupt endocrine function. The World Health Organization (WHO) has linked phthalates to reproductive health concerns globally.

TOXIC CANDLES AND FUMES

Toxic Ingredients:

- **Paraffin Wax:** A petroleum by-product that releases harmful chemicals when burned.

- **Lead-Core Wicks:** Though banned in some regions, lead wicks are still found in certain imports, releasing toxic lead fumes.

- **Artificial Fragrances:** These often contain volatile organic compounds (VOCs) like toluene and benzene.

Harmful Effects:

- **Respiratory Issues:** VOCs and soot from paraffin candles can irritate airways and exacerbate conditions like asthma.

- **Neurological and Developmental Damage:** Lead exposure is linked to cognitive impairments and developmental delays in children.

- **Carcinogenic Risks:** Benzene and toluene are classified as carcinogens and can accumulate in indoor air.

The American Lung Association highlights the dangers of paraffin candles, citing that burning them can emit similar toxins to diesel fuel. A 2009 South Carolina State University study confirmed the presence of carcinogens in paraffin wax fumes.

SUNSCREEN

Toxic Ingredients:

- **Oxybenzone:** A common UV filter linked to hormone disruption.

- **Octinoxate:** Another UV filter, which can alter thyroid function.

- **Retinyl Palmitate:** A form of vitamin A that can produce free radicals when exposed to sunlight.

Harmful Effects:

- **Hormonal Imbalances:** Oxybenzone mimics estrogen, potentially leading to fertility issues and developmental concerns.

- **Skin Damage:** Retinyl palmitate may accelerate skin damage under UV light, paradoxically increasing cancer risk.

- **Environmental Harm:** These chemicals also harm marine ecosystems, particularly coral reefs.

A 2018 study published in the *Journal of the American Medical Association (JAMA)* found that active sunscreen ingredients like oxybenzone enter the bloodstream at levels exceeding safety thresholds within twenty-four hours of application.

RECOMMENDATIONS FOR SAFER ALTERNATIVES

These everyday swaps can significantly reduce exposure to harmful chemicals, protecting both personal health and the environment.

1. **Plastic Food Containers and Utensils:** Opt for glass or stainless-steel containers and wooden utensils.

2. **Candles:** Choose beeswax candles with cotton or wooden wicks.

3. **Sunscreen:** Use mineral-based options with zinc oxide or titanium dioxide as active ingredients. I personally do not use any sunscreen ever. I will wear the appropriate cotton clothing to cover exposed areas during extreme sun conditions. I love the sunshine on my skin and the bare earth and sea under my bare feet.

CHAPTER 5

HOME OF
THE FOUR HORSEMEN

More and more people are starting to realize what some of us health nuts have known and been preaching for decades. The biggest food and beverage brands in the world are the home base of the four dark horseman. It's disgusting to see Coke and Pepsi and Gatorade and Wheaties and McDonald's as major sponsors to all major professional sports brands, including the Olympics, as you see in the advertisements all over the screen during game breaks. It's all about the money. Screw the health of the people, right?

The conduct of the food industry, in my opinion and that of many other professionals, has become one of the biggest crimes in human history. It is literally a profit-over-people culture. The big brands that we all know are literally killing people and wreaking havoc on us and our younger generation. It goes far beyond just making cheap chemically produced filler for more profit. They actually manipulate these lab-made toxic additives to addict you to the texture, flavor, and visual dopamine rush, which rewires your brain. Yup, that's what happens when that saliva secretes in your mouth when you are hungry and smell or look at a bag of Doritos or see a McDonald's sign and your mind can instantly taste a Big Mac, fries, and a Coke.

And it doesn't stop here. It spills over far and wide in every direction, including 90% of the foods you see at every grocery store in America. Even the supposed healthy and organic foods are laced with fake sugars, seed oils, and food dyes. It is one of the biggest problems facing our country—the big companies that pose as great brands alongside professional athletes in TV ads. And those star-studded pro athletes? Yeah, the ones that are worth hundreds of millions of dollars? Well, they're not off the hook either—they're complicit in this whole thing. When I see Lebron James and Peyton and Eli Manning in major primetime TV ads pushing potato chips and soda it makes me sick. They get paid millions to look the other way. Where is the integrity of these supposed role models for our youth?

THE MIGHTY AND POWERFUL FOOD AND BEVERAGE INDUSTRY

The five largest multinational food and beverage companies in the world are Coca-Cola, PepsiCo, Nestlé, Mondelēz International, and Anheuser-Busch InBev. Together, they bring in over $300 billion in annualized sales of toxic snacks and drinks. These companies own extensive portfolios of sub-brands and generate significant global revenue. Look at the toxic sub-brands. These are decay-inducing products, all of them. This is part of what *sick and weak* looks like.

The Coca-Cola Company

Annual Revenue: Over $43 billion in 2023.

Brands: More than 500, including Coca-Cola, Fanta, Sprite, and smartwater. Products are sold in over 200 countries.

Market Position and Global Reach: A leader in non-alcoholic beverages, Coca-Cola invests heavily in sustainability and digital innovation to maintain its dominance.

PepsiCo

Annual Revenue: Approximately $84 billion in 2022.

Brands: Owns iconic names like Lay's, Doritos, Cheetos, Gatorade, Mountain Dew, and Quaker.

Market Position and Global Reach: Operates in over 200 countries and territories, catering to diverse consumer demands with a mix of snacks and beverages.

Nestlé

Annual Revenue: Over $90 billion in 2022.

Brands: Includes KitKat, Nespresso, Purina, and Gerber, totaling around 2,000 brands across various categories.

Market Position and Global Reach: Present in 186 countries

Mondelēz International

Annual Revenue: $31.5 billion in 2022.

Brands: Mondelēz specializes in snacks and confectionery and is known for brands like Oreo, Ritz, Cadbury, and Toblerone.

Market Position and Global Reach: Operates in over 150 countries, targeting the growing demand for snacks worldwide.

Anheuser-Busch InBev (AB InBev)

Annual Revenue: $57.8 billion in 2022.

Market Position and Global Reach: Distribution in over 150 countries, a leader in the brewing and alcohol beverage market.

Brands: Includes Budweiser, Stella Artois, and Corona, with a portfolio of over 500 brands.

Specialization: A global brewing leader focusing on innovation and premium offerings.

These companies dominate their respective markets and utilize economies of scale, vast distribution networks, and aggressive marketing to sustain growth in the toxic beverage and snack industry. Together, they represent a significant portion of the global food and beverage industry, influencing consumer trends and preferences across the world. Consuming toxic foods, snacks, and drinks from these dark companies can trigger an avalanche of problems. One of the most damaging is inflammation. This can take quality years off your life, put you into decay and suffering, and eventually kill you prematurely.

FACTORY FOOD VERSUS EARTH FOOD

Think of factory food as the farthest thing away from the local ground, the local small farm, or the wild ocean (not fish farms, which grow fish in highly toxic conditions). The more it's been touched and handled, the more highly processed it is considered to be. It is often full of the substances that opened this section—the four dark horsemen: fake sugar, trans fats, seed oils, toxic water, and other highly toxic shelf-life extenders. To make it worse, the food is then cooked or prepared in seed oils (if deep fried) or on cooktop grills (grills like those in Five Guys, Chipotle, etc., use seed oils). And remember, the actual foods they serve are the mass-produced crops that are sprayed with harsh chemicals (herbicides, pesticides, etc.) that get carried through from the soil to the root, to the leaf, and finally to the actual fruit or vegetable and then right into your body. Yummy.

Shelf-life extenders, or preservatives, are widely used in processed foods to maintain freshness, prevent spoilage, and extend the products' usability. However, several common preservatives have raised concerns due to their harmful effects on human health. Here are three prominent examples:

BHA and BHT
(Butylated Hydroxyanisole and Butylated Hydroxytoluene)

These are synthetic antioxidants used to prevent oils and fats in foods from becoming rancid. While deemed safe in regulated amounts, studies have linked BHA and BHT to endocrine disruption and potential carcinogenic effects. There are also concerns about their impact on neurological function, with some evidence suggesting they may affect sleep and serotonin regulation.

Sodium Benzoate

Commonly used in acidic foods and beverages, like sodas and pickles, sodium benzoate prevents microbial growth. However, when combined with ascorbic acid (vitamin C), it can form benzene, a known carcinogen. Studies also link sodium benzoate to hyperactivity in children and oxidative stress in cells.

TBHQ (Tertiary Butylhydroquinone)

Found in processed snacks and oils, TBHQ prevents oxidation and extends shelf life. While generally recognized as safe in small amounts, research suggests it may contribute to immune system disruption, liver enlargement, and carcinogenic activity with chronic exposure. Additionally, it has been associated with behavioral changes and neurotoxicity in animal studies.

Many synthetic preservatives work by inhibiting microbial growth or oxidation, but they can also disrupt human health by interacting with biological systems. Potential effects include:

- **Cancer risk:** Certain preservatives, like nitrates and nitrites, can convert into carcinogenic nitrosamines during processing or cooking.

- **Hormonal disruption:** Some preservatives mimic or interfere with natural hormone function, impacting endocrine health.

- **Neurological and behavioral effects:** Ingredients like TBHQ and BHA/BHT may influence brain chemistry, leading to anxiety, hyperactivity, or sleep disruption.

HIGH PRODUCTION CROP FARMING

This is a massive subject, and one that, unfortunately, plays a role in the hidden dangers of living in our toxic world. But it needs to at least be mentioned. For the record, I love the farming community. I've been involved with crop-production science. The independent family farms have been placed into a virtual no-win situation that I won't dive into here.

It's by far too vast a topic for this book and goes deep into poisonous agronomy practices. Just remember this—no farms, no future. The corporate demons and certain factions of the political ecosystem are the largest threat to sustainable eco-friendly farm production. It's disgusting.

I have been on farms all over the world, from small to some of the largest on earth. I studied food production, soil agronomy, and plant health with some of the best soil scientists on earth. It is a fascinating field with some of the brightest people I have ever met. I became so fascinated with the production of healthy, nutrient-dense food farming practices that I actually designed a soil product that got awarded a US patent in 2014, as you'll see on the next page. I designed the first organic, naturally engineered soil that was void of any toxic chemical additives and was totally self-sustaining without any additional minerals needed throughout the plant's entire life cycle, from seed to harvest. And it grows huge lush green plants without the need for any fertilizer. I know a fair amount about healthy, nutrient-dense food production and soil science. I pray to God that it comes back around and starts to gain traction for the good of society.

Healthy, nutrient-dense vegetables and fruits start with healthy, balanced soil that has been properly mineralized. The world's soils used on large production crops have been burned out and destroyed by cheap chemical inputs—mostly NPK (nitrogen, phosphorus, and potassium), which are by-products of fossil fuel production. Unbalanced, chemically fed soils have weaknesses that are a breeding ground for infestation. Natural, healthy, balanced soils (my patent) have very little infestation, if any at all. They are rich in minerals and nutrients, beneficial microorganisms, and organic matter, creating an optimal environment for robust plant growth. Plants grown in such soils develop healthy tissues that are biochemically superior, often containing longer carbon chains in their compounds, such as cellulose, lignin, and other structural components.

These healthy longer carbon chains are more complex and tougher for insects and pests to digest. Since many pests rely on simpler sugars and compounds found in weaker, stressed, or malnourished plants, they tend to avoid healthy plants with these tougher tissues. Furthermore, healthy plants have stronger immune responses, producing secondary metabolites (e.g., phenolics, alkaloids, and terpenes) that help deter pests and inhibit infestations.

In essence, organically balanced soils support the natural resilience of plants, reducing the likelihood of pest attacks and ensuring sustainable, thriving ecosystems.

Sick, weak plants are more vulnerable to pests and infestations because they produce short-chain carbon compounds in their tissues—mainly simple sugars and amino acids. These are easy for insects and pathogens to digest and feed on. In essence, strong plants create tissues that pests can't digest—weak plants become food.

So what does Big Ag do? Here we go again—they cause the problem with chemical fertilizer inputs that grow weak, unstable crops, and then they sell the remedy, herbicides and pesticides to kill the infestation caused by weak plants that can't defend naturally themselves. Monsanto, Bayer, and all the gigantic ag/pharma companies make billions off this process. Sick plants make big money. Sick plants also make sick humans, and sick humans are a much larger profit center over fifty years of hospital visits and drug prescriptions than healthy ones. It is a vicious cycle that is a major part of the problem that makes humans sick and weak. *This is an invisible component of decay* that society unfortunately isn't aware of.

This is why I urge and teach all my clients to support and buy from small local farms. It is just too tough and nearly impossible to avoid the toxic food supply when you buy from the grocery stores that import a large amount of their produce from foreign countries that are largely unmonitored. I have been on some of the largest commercial organic berry farms in the world doing soil testing and tissue sampling and seen the supposed organic fields with my own eyes. Literally miles and miles of rows in each direction. As far as the eye can see. Guess what? They are not organic.

‖ ‖‖‖‖‖‖‖‖‖‖‖‖‖‖‖‖‖‖‖‖‖‖‖‖‖ ‖‖‖‖‖‖‖‖ ‖‖‖‖‖‖‖‖‖‖‖‖ ‖‖‖‖‖‖‖‖ ‖‖‖‖‖‖‖
US008911525Bl

(12) **United States Patent**
Ward

(10) **Patent No.:** **US 8,911,525 Bl**
(45) **Date of Patent:** **Dec. 16, 2014**

(54) **ENGINEERED SOILLESS PLANT CULITVATION MEDIUM**

(71) Applicant: **Nano Growth Technologies, LLC,** Portsmouth, NH (US)

(72) Inventor: **Timothy Ward,** Rye, NH (US)

(73) Assignee: **Nano Growth Technologies, LLC,** Portsmouth, NH (US)

(*) Notice: Subject to any disclaimer, the term of this patent is extended or adjusted under 35 U.S.C. 154(b) by O days.

(21) Appl. No.: **13/913,843**

(22) Filed: Jun.10,2013

(51) **Int. Cl.**
C0SF 11104 (2006.01)
C0SDJ/00 (2006.01)
C05D3/00 (2006.01)
C0SD 5100 (2006.01)
C0SD 9/00 (2006.01)
C0SD 9102 (2006.01)
C0SB 17102 (2006.01)

(52) **U.S. Cl.**
CPC **C0SB 17102** (2013.01)
USPC **71/32**; 71/24; 71/31; 71/33; 71/48; 71/53; 71/63

(58) **Field of Classification Search**
USPC 71/11-63
See application file for complete search history.

(56) **References Cited**

U.S. PATENT DOCUMENTS

3,582,312 A 6/1971 Colectal.
3,990,963 A * 11/1976 Audibert et al 208/179
4,067,716 A * l/1978 Sterrett 71/24
4,074,997 A * 2/1978 Cohen 71/24

4,168,962 A 9/1979 Lambeth
4,174,957 A * 11/1979 Webb etal. 71/24
4,229,442 A * 10/1980 Pinckard 424/725
4,767,440 A * 8/1988 Salac 71/23
5,578,210 A 11/1996 Klecka
5,867,937 A * 2/1999 Templeton 47/59 R
5,900,038 A 5/1999 Wilhelm et al.
5,997,602 A * 12/1999 Aijala.................................... 71/28
6,074,988 A 6/2000 King etal.
7,726,069 Bl 6/2010 Zauche et al.
8,425,819 B2 * 4/2013 Zheng 264/148
8,568,505 B2 * 10/2013 Wells 71/23
8,702,833 B2 * 4/2014 Sugiyama 71/24
8,756,862 Bl* 6/2014 Huberman et al.............. 47/59 S
2003/0089152 Al * 5/2003 Yelanich et al..................... 71/23
2005/0178177 Al 8/2005 Parent et al.

(Continued)

FOREIGN PATENT DOCUMENTS

WO 2007/059583 * 5/2007

OTHER PUBLICATIONS

Boodley, James W. et al., Cornell Peat-Lite Mixes for Commercial Plant Growing, Information Bulletin 43, A Cornell Cooperative Extension Publication, pp. 1-8, 050/100, Revised 4182, Sl. 5M 8008.

(Continued)

Primary Examiner - Wayne Langel
(74) *Attorney, Agent, or Firm* - Andrus Intellectual Property Law LLC

(57) **ABSTRACT**

An engineered soilless plant cultivation medium for potting applications includes specific balanced amounts of nutrient additives. Major nutrient cations (Ca, Mg, K, Na, H) are balanced according to optimal base saturation percentage ranges. Nutrient levels, namely, the amount of major nutrient cations, major nutrient anions and minor nutrients satisfy desired ranges for both standard Mehlich III soil extraction tests and saturated paste tests.

18 Claims, 3 Drawing Sheets

FACTORY FOOD:
MORE WEAPONS OF MASS DESTRUCTION

A diet high in sugar and processed foods is a major contributor to the health crisis in the United States. It has been linked to a number of chronic health conditions, such as obesity, diabetes, heart disease, and certain types of cancer.

According to the CDC, more than two-thirds of adults in the United States are overweight or obese. Obesity is a major risk factor for a number of chronic health conditions, including diabetes, heart disease, and certain types of cancer. The WHO also estimates that diabetes affects around 34 million Americans, and it is one of the leading causes of death in the United States. I suspect this number is low compared to the reality.

The average American consumes around seventeen teaspoons of added sugar per day, which is well above the recommended amount of no more than six teaspoons per day for women and nine teaspoons per day for men. Processed foods, such as frozen dinners and packaged snacks, are often high in added sugars, sodium, and unhealthy fats. Furthermore, a diet high in sugar and processed foods also contributes to heart disease. Consuming added sugar, especially fake sugars, leads to weight gain and dramatically increases risk of heart disease.

A diet high in sugar and processed foods (that contain *all* the dark horsemen, plus more) is a major contributor to the health crisis in the United States. Consuming too much sugar and processed foods has been linked to a number of chronic health conditions, such as obesity, diabetes, heart disease, and certain types of cancer. The average American consumes around seventeen teaspoons of added sugar per day, which is well above the recommended amount, and processed foods are often high in added sugars, sodium, trans fats, fake sugars, and chemical extenders. It is important to limit the intake of all this garbage found in processed foods and to have a balanced diet that includes a variety of earth foods—fruits, vegetables, good fats, and whole proteins.

CHAPTER 6

SEDENTARY LIFESTYLE HEALTH CRISIS

A sedentary lifestyle is characterized as a lack of physical activity and prolonged sitting, which is another major contributor to the health crisis in the United States. According to the US Department of Health and Human Services, nearly 80% of adults do not meet the recommended guidelines for physical activity and more than half of Americans spend at least six hours a day sitting.

This lifestyle choice has been linked to a number of health risks, including obesity, diabetes, heart disease, and certain types of cancer. Sitting for long periods of time has also been associated with a higher risk of early death. Additionally, a sedentary lifestyle can lead to muscle weakness and poor balance, which can increase the risk of falls and injuries, particularly in older adults.

Health risks are compounded by the fact that many Americans have sedentary jobs and spend their leisure time engaging in sedentary activities, such as watching television or surfing social media for hours, or even worse, drinking excessive amounts of alcohol. Talk about decay.

ALCOHOL: A SILENT EPIDEMIC

Please take an honest look at your own alcohol consumption. Excessive alcohol consumption is a silent epidemic that continues to plague millions of Americans. Nearly 55% of US adults report drinking alcohol, with 26% engaging in binge drinking (defined as consuming five or more drinks on a single occasion). The issue is particularly prevalent among young adults aged 18–34, with binge drinking rates reaching 40%, but it spans across all age groups.

Research shows that excessive drinking costs Americans roughly $249 billion annually in lost productivity, healthcare expenses, law enforcement, and other social consequences, equating to over $2.5 billion per day. Many individuals spend hundreds of dollars per month on alcohol, often without realizing the severe toll it takes on their health and well-being.

If you are truly looking to take control of your health and longevity, you need to cut alcohol out of your equation, or at least seriously limit it. It's a simple black dog-white dog decision. Alcohol is a toxin that, over time, ravages multiple organs and systems. Chronic consumption is linked to a range of devastating diseases, including liver cirrhosis, heart disease, pancreatitis, and certain types of cancer (liver, mouth, throat). It also negatively impacts brain function, impairing cognitive abilities and memory while increasing the risk of mental health disorders, including depression and anxiety. Excessive alcohol use also weakens the immune system, making the body more vulnerable to infections.

Ultimately, alcohol is poison to the human body, and its regular consumption can lead to irreversible damage and a significantly reduced quality of life. The harsh reality is that the longer someone drinks excessively, the greater the likelihood of experiencing chronic health issues, early aging, and even premature death.

If you're serious about protecting your health and longevity, it's crucial to recognize alcohol for what it truly is: a slow poison that you can and should avoid or limit to safeguard your vitality.

NO MATTER HOW YOU SLICE IT

Sad but true—America, the richest and most advanced nation in the world, is growing sicker and weaker by the year. Just look at the charts and statistics and numbers. This decline is *not* isolated to any class of person. It crosses all income levels from poor to wealthy, with the poor taking the brunt of its destruction.

It's puzzling to me that a person in the top 10% of wealth status who has the financial means to incorporate comprehensive and qualified fitness and wellness experts and professionals into their lifestyle *won't*. Many are utterly clueless about what they are doing, if anything at all, or haven't a clue on how to measure the quality of who they are choosing to manage their wellness protocols. They have their lives together in so many ways when it comes to finances, legal trusts and wills, asset protection, etc., but they get an F on their fitness and wellness report card. Either they snub their noses because they think they know it all, or they lack the knowledge to choose wisely and have an insufficient perception of what *good* fitness really is.

The flip side is that when they gain insight into the proper protocols of all the touchpoints of what we call The FITNESS QUADRANT, they become obsessed with the reality of how it all links together. They start to see how it can impact their lives dramatically and help them achieve the successful outcomes they are accustomed to in other parts of their lives.

And then pharmaceuticals—oh boy—a drug for this, a drug for that. Watch TV for one hour on a major network and witness it for yourself. America is one of only two countries in the world that allows drug companies to advertise on TV and radio. Imagine that. All the drug commercials that are like expertly crafted Hollywood miniseries to be so seductive to the consumer, convincing tens of millions of uneducated and unsuspecting citizens that they have a condition they didn't even know they had.

But you can call the doctor and get that script. There goes the money train, and there goes the slide into further decay and catabolic despair. And what's the answer when more issues start to appear for that unsuspecting person who started taking the drug? More drugs, baby.

We've got other things that will help you out. Just come on in and get a few more scripts. Wow.

There is not a drug in the world that could ever replace legitimate fitness and nutrition practices and protocols. *Ever.*

IT'S NOT YOUR FAULT

As I leave my house at 5:30 a.m. on the way to the gym to train with several private clients, many thoughts are swirling in my mind. I am obsessed with helping them reach their goals, but my tactic is different than just grinding workouts in the gym. That is unsustainable. I am obsessed with educating my clients so they can become knowledgeable. Knowledge creates success, and success creates sustainability. That is value.

As I weave through traffic, my thoughts center around delivering stellar customized workouts this morning and which issues I need to address with each client pertaining to their goals, health problems, past injuries, etc. I am consumed with thoughts of connecting with them and delivering another invaluable workout that pushes them further into the top-tiered health and strength and wholeness that they have set out to achieve. This is personal for me.

I think about how fortunate I have been to have been exposed to incredible scientific information and the gift I have been given by God to coach, share, and demonstrate this information, which ultimately makes my clients' lives stronger and better. I think about the people around them that look up to them—spouses, children, siblings, elderly parents, close friends, co-workers. I think about the example they are setting for those people, and I am proud of them for committing to a proper fitness routine and sticking with it to make changes to their own health and wellness goals. And in the beginning of their journey with me, about thirty days in, and certainly by the time they are a few months into consistent workouts, cardio bouts, and targeted nutrition, *it* happens. The comments start coming in from their circle of friends and family: "What are you doing? You look really good." "Are you on a diet?" "You look 20 pounds lighter!" "You look really toned." "I've been going to Planet Fitness for seven years. Why can't I get results like that?"

Now things have changed in their minds. Now they are starting to get it, they are on the inside of proper fitness and the front edge of a whole new journey of true health and wellness…without the injuries or starving themselves or spending nine hours in a gym pretending to work out. Ultimately, they are setting the tone for those around them and explaining to their loved ones how important it is to take care of themselves, sparking their interest to do the same. Yeah, show the light to everyone around you by example first. That's it. Influence them to be stronger, healthier, and happier. Because, after all, healthier is happier. And a society of healthy, strong people makes a strong community, region, and country. But it all starts with us. Let's make America healthy and strong. You in?

After thirty-five years of coaching high-level fitness, nutrition, and wellness, I have come to realize I have a job that is extremely important in society. However, I also realize I have a job that I love and hate at the same time. Society has placed you in a losing position when it comes to wellness, fitness routines, etc. Sorry to write this, but 95% of you have been ill informed about how to pursue strength, wellness, and fitness. Dead wrong. No way to win. Virtually no way of achieving big levels of sustainable strength gains or noticeable health and longevity increases. This book is *your* solution if you care to read it, follow it, and act on this information. You have been programmed, manipulated, and misinformed about what's really healthy and how to really get fit.

I heard an amazing quote once:

"IT'S OK TO BE WRONG; BUT IT'S *NOT OK TO STAY WRONG.*"

You are at war, in a battle to stay fit and healthy in a mega-toxic environment. But you don't even realize it because it's invisible, hidden from you. To make it worse, you have been fed a misleading dialogue of fitness misinformation, toxic foods, and loads and loads of pharmaceuticals that are severely damaging to your health. All to make Wall Street, Big Pharma, and Big Medicine billions and billions of dollars annually. You've been set up. Manipulated. Just look at the numbers. America is losing the fight. You see it when you walk into the grocery store or Rite Aid or Walmart. Look around you. What do you see? Do you see healthy, fit, vibrant people? What do you see on the store shelves? Whole foods that are from the source? Nope. You see rows and rows of chemical-laden processed drinks, snacks, and mass-produced, low-level garbage vitamins and supplements that are virtually all man-made trash.

Welcome to the matrix. Across the world, hundreds of millions of people wake up every morning and start their day with what they call a workout at the gym or at a small group studio. Virtually none of the gym owners give a damn about your workout methods. I know about twenty of them personally. All they really care about is that EFT (electronic funds transfer) every thirty days. Even worse, people are being led by "trainers" who I believe are well intentioned but don't have a clue what they are talking about or how to work out properly. I see it every day. I also know well over fifty of them personally, and for the most part, they are great folks. But the results of these hundreds of millions of people flocking to the gym every day around the world? Look at the statistics. They are *horrifying*. They sustain injuries and have no success, no control, and zero chance at any sustainable personal progress *at all*. Then add in horrible toxic nutrition...*yikes*. Absolute disaster.

WHY?

Have you ever noticed how easy it is to invest in everything *but* our health?

We have a priority problem.

Think about it: we prioritize our expensive cars, five-star chic restaurants every weekend, med-spas, social media profiles, designer watches, shoes, jewelry, and the latest tech. And how about that $300,000 boat you use eleven times a year? We proudly manicure our lawns, upgrade our phones, splurge on vacations, designer clothes, private golf club memberships, and that $8,000 handbag—because it makes a statement, right? And there's nothing wrong with wanting nice things.

But here's the question I invite you to consider: what kind of statement are you making about *you*—your physique, your personal energy, your vitality, your longevity?

It's common to see people spend thousands a month on dining out, entertainment, and luxury upgrades, but when it comes to investing in their health—where it really counts—many hesitate. They put it off. They try shortcuts. Or worse, they assume it's too late to make meaningful changes.

Here's the truth: your body is the one possession you take with you every step of your life. And unlike that car, handbag, or golf membership, your body doesn't come with a trade-in option.

This isn't a guilt trip—it's an invitation. An invitation to reframe what matters most.

Because if we're being honest, climbing the stairs without gasping for air, waking up energized, thinking clearly, and being strong enough to live fully—that's luxury. That's freedom. That's power.

So the challenge isn't about judgment. It's about alignment. Aligning your daily choices with the kind of life you actually want to live— vibrant, mobile, mentally sharp, and strong. Not just now, but ten, twenty, thirty years from now.

It's not about perfection. It's about prioritization.

The world has made it too easy to get sick, weak, and distracted. But that doesn't have to be your story. You can flip the equation. You can choose to prioritize *you*—your real wealth: your body, your brain, your well-being.

Because when you do, everything else in life gets better.

SO WHY SHOULD YOU CARE?

For most of us, the early years feel like a free ride. Up until around age 40, youth has your back. You can bounce back from late nights, overindulgence, and those *friendly* Thanksgiving football games that left you limping for a week—and somehow still recover without much thought. Your body quietly handles the abuse.

But eventually, things shift. You wake up one day and realize your body doesn't bounce back like it used to. The aches last longer. The weight sticks around. Your energy dips. Welcome to what's known as *biological aging*—a gradual, invisible process where your cells, muscles, and systems start losing ground. It's not your fault. It's not punishment. It's nature. But that doesn't mean you're powerless.

Here's the good news: you can take control—if you decide to. The truth is, the body *will* adapt—it just needs a new kind of input. What worked (or didn't) in your twenties won't cut it now. That's not a failure. That's an invitation. You need to recognize the change and act on it.

You've likely had those quiet, personal conversations with yourself. In the car. On a walk. Lying in bed at night.

"I need to lose 40 pounds."

"I should stop drinking."

"I've got to eat better."

"I can't keep ignoring my health."

"My knees hurt just walking upstairs."

"My back's been off for years since high school football."

"I eat salads…why am I still stuck?"

These thoughts aren't weakness. They're signals. And they're common—you're not alone.

Let me share a story. I have a friend who tried a trendy weight-loss program through a popular multi-level marketing company. Every day, she replaced lunch with a meal replacement shake full of artificial ingredients, skipped real food, and saved up all her hunger for a big nightly dinner. She lost 42 pounds—half of it was muscle. For a while, it seemed like it was working.

But eventually…all the weight came back—plus 12 extra pounds and zero muscle. So did the pain. Her lower back started acting up again. Walking became her only option—tracked by a smartphone app that celebrates 10,000 steps. The program promised a shortcut, but shortcuts rarely lead to lasting change.

This is what I want to help you avoid—the cycle of quick fixes, frustration, and starting over. It's an example of the Sisyphean struggle in Section 1. Because the truth is, there *is* a better way. A smarter, more sustainable, and more powerful strategy that doesn't require starving yourself or chasing trends. You just need the right system—one that leverages your biology, accounts for your age, and your untapped potential.

The decisions you make now are the ones that shape how you'll feel five, ten, even twenty years from now.

You're not broken. You're just a little behind. You're just at the crossroads. And you're reading this for a reason.

Let's move forward—stronger, smarter, and on your terms.

CHAPTER 7

SO SMART
THEY'RE STUPID

In the previous section, I made a statement: I realize I have a job that I love and hate at the same time. Here's what I meant by that. Like most of us, I have a pretty robust network of friends. I have built many relationships from being highly active in the community as an athlete, playing several sports, from baseball to basketball to tennis to football, and then from having my own kids—two boys that are my everything, my gifts from God—and coaching them along with hundreds of kids on organized team sports year-round, as well as business friends, etc.

Here's my pain. Several of those friends and acquaintances are struggling, really struggling, with their health, wellness, fitness, and nutrition. It's literally all around me in my personal life. They are out of shape—like 90% of them never get rolling on any legitimate health regimen, and they constantly complain about it, yet they always seem to have all the answers on what to do to lose that belly, gain mobility and strength, etc. It is unbelievable to me the things they attempt and the attitudes they have about their "new eating routine" or "new fitness workout." It's astonishing how utterly blind they are when it comes to fitness and wellness. It is painful for me to see them struggle. I want them to thrive, but they will not listen to the truth.

These are smart and successful people I am referring to. Very accomplished in certain categories of life. They are some of the smartest people I know—much smarter than I am with business or finance or law. But they are absolute morons (like me with some things!) at taking care of themselves through fitness and nutrition protocols. They don't stand a chance for any improvement at all because they don't prioritize it, let alone understand it. The comments they make to me about their fitness regimen and the new diets they are trying are truly sad. They will never achieve any goals they are setting out to achieve with how they are approaching it. *Ever*.

Eventually, the worst always happens. They ask me soft questions about what they are trying—often some kind of fasting thing involving consuming red crushed peppers and lemons every twenty-nine hours. Fasting, fasting, and more fasting because they saw it on YouTube and Instagram and that lady who posted it is hot, so it must be effective! They want to know if their new thing will work. When I begin to provide them with some rock-solid science on things they should consider, they immediately bow out and say, "Well, I can't work out how you and Julie do. I'll just stick with this new routine and my new salad diet." Yup. The "salad" thing again.

YOUR DOOR IS CLOSING

As we get older, something starts to happen quietly and gradually. We don't always notice it right away, but it's real. Our energy dips. Our bounce-back slows. The body that once felt bulletproof doesn't recover like it used to. And by the time we hit 45 or 50, it starts to really show. The door to our younger self begins to close, and if we don't do something about it, it won't open again.

We start to feel the wear and tear—joints ache more, muscle fades faster, and fatigue creeps in quicker than it used to. That old spark we used to take for granted feels harder to find. But here's the deal: this isn't just "getting old." It's the result of neglecting the things that truly keep us strong—our muscle, our movement, our nutrition, and our mindset.

The good news? It's not over. Not even close.

There's a smarter way to age—a system built on resistance training, efficient cardio, and proper nutrition that actually helps you regain strength, energy, and freedom. Top this off with peptide therapy and wow. Here comes a new you. This isn't about chasing vanity or pretending you're 25 again. It's about staying sharp, mobile, capable, and strong enough to live life fully—on your terms.

Muscle isn't just for athletes. It's your armor. It's your engine. It's the difference between independence and dependence as you age.

So here's the truth: the longer you wait, the harder it gets. But right now, you still have a choice. You can take back control. You can rebuild. You can turn the tide.

This is your shot to do something powerful—not out of fear, but out of purpose. Start building the body that will carry you strong into the next ten, twenty, or even thirty years. You've still got chapters left to write—and they can be the strongest ones yet.

WAKE UP EVERYBODY

I love that incredible song "Wake Up Everybody" by the late Teddy Pendergrass both lyrically and musically, and of course, he opens up the golden pipes to bring magic to the recording. But if you understand the message of this masterful tune, he's calling for everyone to wake up to the causes of the day. He's asking people to wake up, saying there's a better way. Pump the brakes on your busy life and wake up.

These legendary words also work for your personal fitness and wellness journey today. This may be your last chance to truly get a grip on your health and actually do something about it. I'm telling you that, as I write this, I truly believe some of you will actually make a decision and realize how much the proper type of lifestyle and fitness can change your trajectory of health and well-being. You see, aging is so sneaky. It compounds as time goes by. And as time goes by, the loss and decline of components vital to our physical body and mental acuity accelerate, and before you know it, you have decayed enough that many new problems are on the rise.

One example of this is muscle loss. Muscle is one of the vital tissues you *cannot* afford to lose. It is a marker of your health and longevity status, as many scientific studies have now shown. These are easy to find—google it and you'll see. I certainly want you to save what muscle you have now, but I actually want you to gain more as well. By doing so, you will automatically start changing your body composition, which is more important than your weight. In basic terms, this is what your body is made up of—a mix of muscles, bones, and fat.

Fat is technically named adipose tissue—the stuff you see on your belly, ass, arms, etc. Then there is visceral and organ fat, the really dangerous stuff inside our bodies that we cannot see. You want to reduce this bad fat along with yellow adipose tissue, which is mostly on your stomach, ass and thighs, lower back, and the back of your arms. And the way that reduction in fat happens is through a combination of some vital pieces—most notably, resistance training, proper nutrition, and cardio work all in combination. The first two pieces are a requirement to build muscle. There is *no* other way you will achieve hypertrophy (muscle growth). That is not my opinion but fact-based science.

As the sun rises on another day, millions of people over the age of 45 find themselves overlooking a vital opportunity that could transform their lives—the power of knowledge and choice. The vast difference between growth and decay. *The GOAT Within* highlights the untapped potential wherein lies a life-changing experience that can bring about a new level of physical and mental well-being, enhancing every aspect of life. However, this happens only if it is done properly! This is and always has been the problem of achieving fitness success. When fitness is proper, the result is a tidal wave of benefits. Rivers of hormonal growth factors are released into the bloodstream during a proper exercise bout, signaling cellular growth (IL-10) and a vast array of anabolic stimulation to your entire body. From increasing muscle mass and improving joint health to restoring mobility and igniting a sense of empowerment, the journey toward living strong and healthy through high-level fitness protocols and nutrition is one that beckons with the indisputable reality of rejuvenation and fulfillment.

As individuals reach middle age, they gradually become resigned to the notion that physical decline is an inevitable part of the aging process. However, the truth is that proper fitness training and nutrition can break these limiting beliefs, unveiling a world of possibilities beyond what was previously deemed possible. The next section serves as a clarion call to everyone over 45, encouraging them to embrace this golden opportunity with unwavering determination and enthusiasm. This is the right way to weave proper fitness into your life.

One of the most striking benefits of engaging in high-level exercises is the significant increase in muscle mass it brings. Muscle mass not only promotes strength and stability but also plays a critical role in elevating the body's metabolism. This increase helps combat the natural slowing of metabolism that often occurs with age, making weight management more achievable. By incorporating strength training routines into their lives, individuals can reclaim their lost muscle mass, fortifying their bodies with an armor of strength that will carry them gracefully through the years. This is where the difference lies—high-quality, adequate resistance training comes with a rock-solid requirement of exercise sciences and knowledge. There is no compromise and no second place. It's black and white.

But fitness transcends mere physicality; it is an inseparable union of the body and mind. As people embark on their fitness journey, they begin to witness a profound transformation in their mental well-being. Exercise has been scientifically proven to release endorphins, the brain's natural mood elevators, fostering a sense of positivity and reducing stress. As physical fitness increases, improved focus and cognitive function become more evident, and the ability to cope with life's challenges becomes more robust. Moreover, an empowered mind enhances the motivation to continue striving toward one's goals, both in fitness and life overall.

Beyond the mental benefits, high-level exercises bring about a remarkable improvement in joint health and integrity. The aging process often brings with it joint discomfort, making movements more rigid and restricted. However, uncompromised proper fitness routines involving strength training, mobility, and flexibility exercises help lubricate the joints (see the section on synovial fluid) and increase their range of motion. As a result, everyday tasks become easier, and the fear of debilitating joint pain dissipates, allowing individuals to regain control of their lives. Just imagine the payoff—moving much easier with strength and balance through everyday tasks. Remember, healthier is happier.

Perhaps one of the most liberating aspects of fitness training is the newfound sense of physical freedom it leads to. As range of motion expands, doors to once-lost passions begin to reopen. Hiking that picturesque trail, dancing with a loved one, or simply bending down to pick up a grandchild become not only possible but also immensely enjoyable experiences. These seemingly small yet profound moments become the building blocks of an enriched and more fulfilling life. It is really true that healthier is happier.

Moreover, the positive effects of proper fitness training and nutrition extend far beyond the physical and mental realms. The benefits cascade into every aspect of daily life, impacting relationships, career aspirations, and overall life satisfaction. As individuals feel more confident in their bodies, they radiate a contagious energy that draws others toward them. This newfound magnetism enhances personal connections and fosters a greater sense of community and belonging. You are just plain stronger in all aspects of your life. How does that sound? Talk about becoming happier!

The journey toward healthy and strong may seem daunting at first, but it is crucial to remember that every endeavor begins with a single step. As the saying goes, "Rome wasn't built in a day," and the same holds true for transforming your life through the GOAT that lies deep inside you. The key is to gain knowledge and access to proper protocols so you know what you are doing. You need 100% clarity on not just *what* to do, but *how* to do it. Then start and remain consistent, for it is the dedication to incremental progress that yields lasting results. The secret to success lies in finding joy in the process, celebrating every milestone, and being compassionate toward yourself during setbacks.

Following legitimate coaching and protocols and partnering with like-minded individuals can provide invaluable support and encouragement along the way. Sharing triumphs and struggles fosters a sense of camaraderie that propels everyone toward success. Age is no barrier to greatness, and fitness partnerships and strong communities exemplify the power of solidarity in achieving transformative life changes. This is why I often advocate for people to team up with a partner to make the journey together—a husband and wife team, two or three best friends, or how about a dad and son or daughter doing some training and cooking together. This is the enriching part of fitness and wellness, which can be central to long-lasting wellness commitments.

The opportunities that await those over 45 through proper fitness training and nutrition are nothing short of life changing. By engaging in high-level exercises, you can increase muscle mass, improve joint health and joint integrity, and unlock a newfound sense of freedom and vitality. Fitness is a holistic journey that transcends the physical, empowering the mind, body, and spirit. It instills a profound sense of purpose and satisfaction, improving every aspect of life, from personal relationships to career endeavors.

So, if you're 45 or older and find yourself questioning whether it's too late to embark on this transformative journey, remember this: age is but a number, and the future remains unwritten, the pages awaiting your pen strokes. The power of proper fitness training and nutrition is a gift that knows no boundaries and bestows upon its recipients the limitless potential for ageless vitality. Embrace this opportunity with open arms, lean into it, and you'll discover that the most extraordinary chapters of your life are possibly yet to be written, fueled by the boundless energy and inspiration that fitness provides. Take the first step today, and let your journey toward a healthier, happier, and more fulfilling life begin. But most of all—*do it the right way*.

SECTION 2 TAKEAWAYS

- Toxic foods sabotage even the best fitness training routines.

- Know the four dark horsemen, how to find them, and avoid them at all costs.

- Fake factory foods, beverages, and snacks need to be 100% removed from your life.

- Make "earth foods" your first and only choice for all your meals and snacks.

- Prioritize learning proper knowledge and then put it into action before your door is closed.

- Learn the proper way to make yourself stronger and then teach your loved ones.

- Stop the daily lifestyle habits that cause inactivity and fitness avoidance.

SECTION 3

LIVING STRONGER, BETTER, AND LONGER

Before we get to the formulas, let's look at the importance of our environment.

Show me your friends, and I'll show you your future. Your social environment matters.

If you happen to have a crew of friends who are into health and fitness, that's fantastic. However, if your friends have poor lifestyle habits and zero interest in getting strong and healthy, maybe it's time to start socializing with some new people who have a passion for living strong and staying healthy?

I'm not saying you should totally abandon your old friends, but there is a tremendous toll people can pay for hanging out with the wrong crowd. The social influence we have on each other can be tremendous, and it works in both directions. So why not gravitate toward healthy-minded individuals who strongly support health and longevity?

There is nothing better than having a group of friends who are passionate about living strongly. That's one thing I love about the gym. Everyone there is seeking to get better and live stronger. What a positive environment to be in for a few hours every week instead of a barroom.

One of the key takeaways from this section is that there is an entry point into fitness at every level, from beginner to professional athlete. Whether you are 53 or 78 years old and have never stepped into a gym, there is an appropriate entry point for you to start in a basic routine. If you are a professional athlete, there is an appropriate entry point into a high-level complex routine. For everybody in between, there is an appropriate entry point into an adequate regimen that will differ from the other two. No matter what your point of entry, properly written protocols will move the needle for you and get you far past the sticking points you are most likely experiencing if you already train, and certainly if you have never worked out before. It's all about knowledge, quality coaching, and professional guidance.

The reality is, we all have different goals, limitations, expectations, opinions, and reasons we do things. When it comes to health routines and working out, fitness science narrows the field on these individual topics, and the road to effective fitness becomes very narrow. You have to choose wisely. Legitimate exercise science matters, and it is vitally important to adhere to it in order to properly trigger the right systems and functions so that they will respond appropriately (growth and repair). Remember, a poor stimulus leads to poor results and vice versa. This is 100% indisputable. Living strong is never achieved with singular or inadequate activity. It is always a four-phase combination, a.k.a. The FITNESS QUADRANT. *Always*.

Living strong means connecting the proper pieces of fitness, nutrition, cardiovascular training, and recovery all together in a synergistic format. You can have the greatest strength workouts in the world, but if your nutrition is inadequate (or toxic!), you'll never fully capitalize on the benefits of that training. Additionally, if your heart and lungs are not routinely trained and maintained, your cardiovascular health will suffer, and even worse, will rapidly begin to decline after the age of 45. Lastly, if you are a gung-ho extremist who has harmful stimuli (awful exercise form, etc.) and inadequate recovery periods, you will be on a one-way road to Injury-Ville.

There is a way to execute resistance training movements that are *scientifically correct and superior*. There is a nutritional requirement of whole protein intake to support protein synthesis (muscle growth and repair, joint integrity, etc.) that is *scientifically correct*. There is a formula for cardiovascular protocols—a certain heart rate zone that burns the most body fat and strengthens the heart and lungs—that is also *scientifically correct*. And there is a required optimal recovery period that is also *scientifically* correct. No matter your age or your physical condition (other than physical incapacitations), whether you are 16 years old or 83 years old, the cold hard facts remain. Muscle contracts the same way, muscle needs whole proteins to repair and grow, your heart and lungs strengthen or weaken the exact same way, and you need appropriate recovery periods to reap the rewards of growth (living stronger) and avoid decay (living sick and weak).

CHAPTER 1

MUSCLE IS MAGIC

Before I share the badass blueprint that helps you live stronger, better, and longer, you'll need to understand more about the muscle mass on your body, how vitally important it is, and how to add more of it properly. This is one of the most important takeaways for you from this book.

A muscle cell requires seven times more energy than a fat cell. The fewer muscle cells you have, the lower your caloric burn rate, which means more fat on your body. The greater your muscle volume (lean body mass), the higher your caloric burn rate, meaning less fat on your body. Learn how to add muscle to your frame if you want to burn more calories/fat 24/7 and become lean.

This striking image below shows a side by side visual of the same body weight female but how much larger her body is with a higher percentage of body fat compared to a leaner, tighter, more muscular body at the same weight. It shows how much denser muscle is than fat (yellow adipose tissue). Muscle is truly magic, and you need to keep it on your body at all costs, especially as you age.

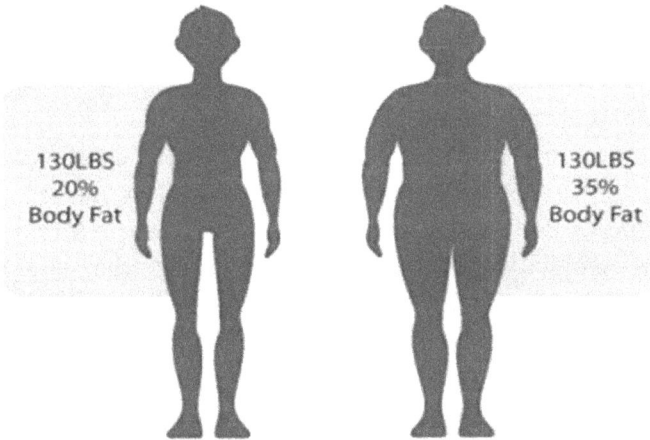

THINK FAT LOSS
NOT WEIGHT LOSS

130LBS
20%
Body Fat

130LBS
35%
Body Fat

The more muscle you have, the more fat you burn, the slimmer you look

MUSCLE MASS BY THE YEARS

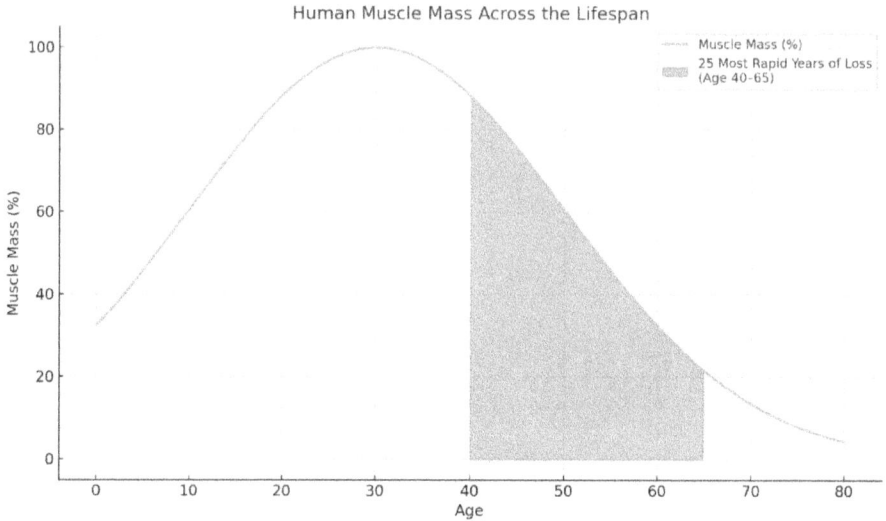

Human Muscle Mass Across the Lifespan

As you can see, our greatest loss of muscle occurs between age 40 through approximately 65 years old. This is why these years are the most vital for having a legitimate strategy to stop the loss. Multiple research studies undeniably conclude muscle mass is a major marker and key to longevity. Another key driver and marker is strength, as you'll see on the chart below. Strength is a derivative of muscle. If you lose your muscle, you lose your strength, then you lose your ability to move efficiently. The graphs show the losses are virtually identical. You then start to overcompensate for your lack of strength, thus setting up a host of imbalances that trigger injuries, which set in and grow at an exponential rate.

You cannot age strong and live strong on this path. Your answer to reversing the loss of muscle and strength and the beginning of gaining muscle and strength is resistance training practiced in a very particular way.

Human Strength Across the Lifespan

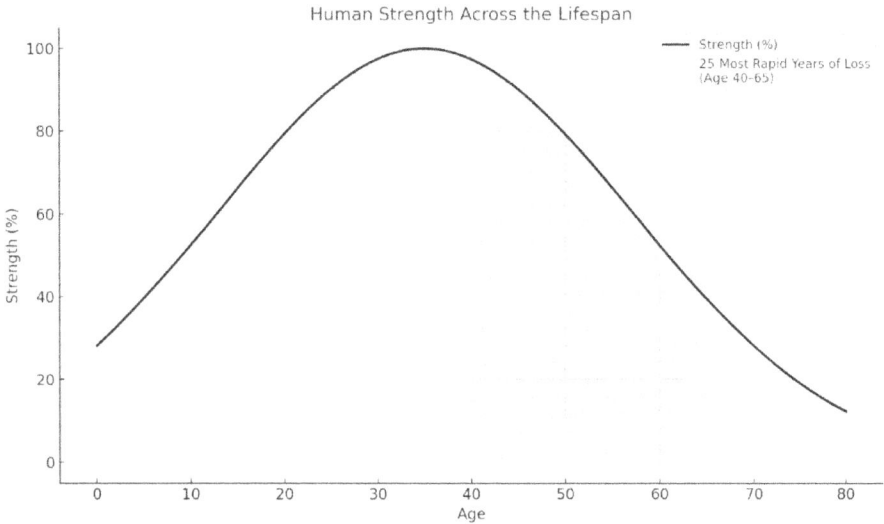

REVERSE THESE TWO EQUATIONS

What triggers muscle growth and increases in strength (hypertrophy)?

Resistance training consists of strength exercises that happen in a variety of ways with a cross section of different equipment like barbells, dumbbells, kettlebells, cable machines, plate-loaded machines, bodyweight, rubber bands, heavy balls, etc. It is without a doubt the most complex and the most misunderstood form of training, and by far the most misused in the entire fitness space. The complexities of resistance training are far-reaching and go very deep into exercise sciences.

The most egregious offenders against proper resistance exercise are the large majority of traditional medical doctors and the far-out, hardcore workout extremists who think they know it all yet have zero formal training. They are often injured, sometimes so severely that surgery is the only remedy. With the exception of a few, virtually all conventional medical doctors are grossly incompetent when it comes to exercise physiology, how to implement proper protocols, and what it really means to strength train properly. The classic advice doctors often dole out to patients is, "Go lift some weights. Yeah, you need to do some strengthening exercises." And that's it. It ends there. No guidance, no strategies, no plan. Just go strength train.

It's not really their fault. They are virtually all trained to manage sickness, prescribe drugs, and make bank from the large pharmaceutical companies. Perhaps this is why many traditionally trained medical doctors are opening their own private practices where they can implement solutions to healing as well as true fitness and nutrition platforms and protocols. This allows them to focus on preemptive and preventive measures to get healthy and stay healthy. Remember, more drugs equals more problems.

WHY RESISTANCE TRAINING IS SUPERIOR VS. POPULAR FITNESS WORKOUTS

There's no getting around it. If your ultimate goal is building more muscle mass—the single most important longevity marker—you cannot rely on yoga, Pilates, spin classes, or even high-intensity boot camps like Orange Theory. Are these workouts bad? Absolutely not. They can improve flexibility, boost cardiovascular fitness, and burn calories. For many people, they serve a purpose. But let's be clear— they are not designed to build muscle and they never will, and without adding more muscle, you cannot pushback or reverse the inevitable decline of aging.

Resistance training, especially when executed through MIT protocols using dumbbells, kettlebells, Olympic bars, cable systems, TRX bands, and a large spectrum of commercial gym equipment, stands in a category of its own. These tools provide the exercise variety, progression, adequate resistance, and biomechanical precision needed to fully stimulate the body's muscle and muscle chains and trigger hypertrophy across the entire musculoskeletal system. There are 640 major muscles in the human body that require proper targeting to trigger muscle growth. These various popular fitness workouts do not come close to accomplishing this. Proper resistance training is the direct solution for the aging process: more muscle, more strength, more protection for your bones, stronger joints, increased metabolism, higher level of hormone production, and more energy.

So yes, spin, yoga, Pilates, and Orange Theory can be fine add-ons. Terrific side dishes. In fact, I recommend yoga to my more muscular clients to improve their flexibility. But they're not the foundation. They are not the main dish. Resistance training is the foundation. It's the king of fitness modalities because it alone builds the structural armor in all 640 major muscles that determines whether you age strong, capable, and youthful, or whether you slide into weakness, fragility, and declining muscle mass.

RESISTANCE TRAINING VS. POPULAR FITNESS TRENDS

Category	Yoga / Pilates / Spin / Orange Theory	MIT Resistance Training
Primary Goal	Flexibility, calorie burn, cardiovascular fitness, stress reduction	Building muscle mass (top longevity marker), strength, metabolic health, cardio endurance, anabolic triggers
Muscle Growth (Hypertrophy)	*Minimal to none—* not designed to create new muscle tissue	*Direct and significant—* targets full muscle chains for measurable hypertrophy; adequate loads for adaptive remodeling of muscle
Exercise Options	Limited variations, mostly bodyweight or cardio-based	Vast selection: dumbbells, kettlebells, Olympic bars, cables, TRX, vast amount of machines, bodyweight, plyometrics
Biomechanics	Low resistance, not enough load to	Precision mechanics with progressive resistance that

Category	Yoga / Pilates / Spin / Orange Theory	MIT Resistance Training
	stimulate structural adaptation	forces the body to adapt and grow
Longevity Impact	Helps with mobility, balance, and cardio health	Directly combats aging by preserving and increasing muscle mass—the #1 longevity marker; improves mobility, balance, and bone density
Metabolism & Fat Loss	Burns calories during the workout	Builds lean muscle that burns calories 24/7, raising metabolic rate long term
Structural Protection	Improves posture and flexibility	Builds "armor" for bones, joints, and connective tissue; true protection against frailty
Best Use	Acceptable add-on for mobility, recovery, or enjoyment	Non-negotiable foundation of lifelong strength, vitality, and youthfulness

THE FITNESS QUADRANT: YOUR BADASS BLUEPRINT

The FITNESS QUADRANT is a master system. It is your ticket to aging super strong and healthy. Muscle, strength, mobility, a strong heart, lungs, and circulatory system, longevity, and well-being is the payoff. It's a superior system and a master road map for understanding the combination of the four phases of high-level effective fitness that trigger the anabolic growth mode *that keeps you young*. It is applicable to everyone, from professional athletes to people in their 80s looking for strength, mobility, and coordination (balance) improvements.

Build The FITNESS QUADRANT system into your life to live healthy and strong:

- **Avoid toxic foods and products:** these destroy your vital systems.

- **Resistance exercise**: this is your muscle stimulus to gain and maintain muscle.

- **Nutrition choices**: make earth food and whole proteins a priority to repair tissue.

- **Cardiovascular work**: a strong circulatory system (heart and lungs) is gold.

- **Recovery**: Recharge your battery, mentally relax and enjoy yourself.

- **Get a posse:** keep a circle of true friends to build positive vibes and mental connectivity.

Each quadrant has its own ecosystem and own scientific framework. When all four are properly executed, then linked together in a weekly plan, that magic formula I mentioned in the introduction begins to deliver major progress and success. And one of the best parts is you get fit in half the normal time because the four quadrants together hit triggers that begin to pull metrics out of your physiology that skyrocket your growth. Your fitness and longevity plan should not dominate your weekly schedule if it is done properly, but it should dominate your priorities if you want to live in strength and growth and not in weakness and decay.

FITNESS QUADRANT®

RESISTANCE

R

Builds/Maintains Muscle Mass
Joint Health & Mobility

NUTRITION

N

Tissue Repair Essentials
Energy & Metabolism

CARDIO

C

Strong Heart & Lungs
Lower Blood Pressure

RECOVERY

R

Recharge & Repair
Neurological Growth
(neurogenesis)

- The four quadrants all work together. It is complete fitness.
- Top left quadrant "R" is the most complex and most important.
- Left side of the quadrant is active. Right side is passive.

LIFE STRONG
HEALTHIER IS HAPPIER

A master professional system, our trademarked FITNESS QUADRANT not only helps you understand the difference between the four major phases of fitness and what those specific phases address but how to combine them in a format that meets *your* individualized goals or intended outcomes based on your unique situation. It applies to beginners, professional athletes, and everyone in between that are interested in building their own fitness, wellness, or performance ecosystem.

As an example, a pro athlete who is going for a $200 million contract and is in a sport that requires explosive directional change movements, power, speed, and endurance will spend more time in the upper left R quadrant and lower left quadrant, performing specific resistance movements that build motor unit recruitment patterns that mimic their specific sport. Additionally, the speed and endurance portion will be performed at a level that mimics the cardiovascular loading requirements specific to the performance patterns during competition. The upper right nutrition quadrant will be adjusted to supply adequate macronutrients (protein, carbs, and lipids) to accommodate the energy expenditure and adequate complete protein levels that account for protein turnover and hypertrophy. The lower right quadrant, recovery, is important for everyone, and it is mostly overlooked, especially by high-level athletes who become victims of overtraining. Mixed Martial Arts (UFC) athletes are a prime example. They are so driven and determined that they sometimes overtrain and actually start sliding backwards and, unfortunately, open the door to a higher probability of injury.

On the other end of the spectrum, if someone in their mid 60s or 70s has a hard time getting up and down stairs or off a couch, the training regimen will also focus on the upper left quadrant (resistance), but the modalities will be focused on progressive strength movements for the hip, glute, lower back, quads, and hamstrings. Additional emphasis on mobility, balance, and stability triggers taps into the central nervous system by initiating and increasing motor unit recruitment efficiencies (muscle firing) and collapsing multi-muscle chain reaction times, body position, movement coordination, and balance, called proprioception.

The four quadrants all work together in combination. Each quadrant has a drop-down list that dives into the important components of that quadrant. Implement The FITNESS QUADRANT system and you will rapidly gain muscle, strength, energy, and a vitality that is undeniable.

THE FOUR PHASES OF THE FITNESS QUADRANT

R = RESISTANCE
(top left quadrant)

This is where muscle is built. Resistance training is the master trigger that unlocks all the other quadrants at many levels to unleash a tidal wave of benefits and growth factors. It is important to understand that, according to the goal of the average individual, fitness enthusiast, or competitive athlete, there are many different variations, and thus different modalities of training necessary to achieve the desired outcome. As an example, a sprinter or shot put athlete trains in a completely different mode than a long-distance runner, triathlete, or tennis player. For most individuals seeking fitness, the most pursued goal is typically to gain muscle and strength, lose and manage fat, or gain cardiovascular endurance. In our case with our clients, we also look to gain flexibility, mobility, joint strength, and to increase balance and stability. These are all achievable through resistance training modalities and systems, regardless of your body type.

Resistance training is the king of fitness. It's the biggest bang for your buck when it comes to replenishing your physical currency and adding *multiple vital pieces* to your quality of life and longevity. Unfortunately, because of its complexity, it is also the most misunderstood and the most "hacked" part of fitness for many reasons.

Here are four vital factors that are a requirement for strength and hypertrophy gains:

1. Adequate resistance on muscle chains

2. Understanding weight selection and synchronous versus asynchronous firing patterns

3. Understanding the role of proper biomechanics (form) on motor unit firing and safety

4. Understanding the role of ATP-PC bioenergetics formula

These four factors are the exact reason elite athletes, and a few elite trainers, get the most out of their training programs in the R quadrant.

Assuming your exercise form (biomechanics) is correct, one of the most important principles of stimulating muscle growth is choosing the proper weight to exercise with.

You must understand this. There has to be adequate stress on the muscle in order to trigger hypertrophy (muscle growth).

As a rule of thumb, a rep range between 6 and 15 should be the target. It means that your 6th or 15th rep should be a major struggle to complete with perfect form, and it would be impossible to do one more rep. That's the right weight selection.

A large majority of gym participants never reach their goals because of this one principal alone. Of course, there are many more reasons. However, this is a requirement above everything else.

Understanding your weight selection matters to your success for muscle gains.

Additionally, if you are brand new to strength training, starting with a weight that is above these ranges is completely fine so you can understand the proper form.

Once this is achieved, increasing the amount of resistance will be critical for strength and muscle gains, as mentioned above.

When we say muscle is magic, we really mean that muscle is the primary pathway to health and longevity. And we mean resistance training is the only stimulus that will drive protein synthesis (hypertrophy). Just eating healthy *does not* stimulate muscle growth. This does not discount the value of nutrition or cardiovascular training one bit. They too are vital pieces of superior fitness programming. It means that there are many more triggers that get activated when resistance training is done properly.

Resistance makes your nutrition and your cardio performance all that much better. After resistance training bouts, your body is in overdrive for nutritional support, especially in the first 45 minutes after training, when glycogen uptake is at a peak and when you can turn off the catabolic engine and turn on the anabolic engine. This 45-minute window after your workout is an important time slot in your nutritional timing. The proper nutrition (liquid supplement immediately after a training bout) will take you out of a catabolic state—which you're in for several hours after training—and place you in an anabolic state. Furthermore, certain higher rep range resistance training bouts trigger systems in your body that increase capillary density and mitochondrial density, thus increasing aerobic capacity and adenosine triphosphate and creatine phosphate (ATP-CP) storage.

In other words, you can eat a pristine diet 24/7 and do cardio until your respiratory system is at peak performance, but neither of these two pieces will ever maintain or build muscle in the human body. In fact, a dominating cardiovascular fitness routine will actually take muscle *off* the body through a process called gluconeogenesis—a muscle breakdown process that converts certain amino acids found in muscle to glycogen. During gluconeogenesis, muscle is broken down into amino acids, which are pushed through the liver for conversion into the energy source glycogen used to fuel your cardio bouts. So, eating a fantastic diet is great and essential, but it will not adequately build muscle on the human frame. Properly performed resistance training is the only stimulus that will trigger hypertrophy.

Adequate Resistance

Adequate resistance is needed in order to force an adaptive response for muscle growth. This means you cannot grab 5-pound dumbbells and do 45 curls to "feel the burn" and expect to get the benefit of hypertrophy. That is simply not enough resistance to trigger an adaptive response. Period. There is no reason—*zero*—for the body to react to that stimulus because it is not enough resistance to cause physical and biological triggers of muscle growth (synchronous versus asynchronous muscle fiber firing). This, along with incorrect form, is by far the biggest problem for people trying to make gains in their strength, wellness, and longevity, and they never achieve any of these intended outcomes. It is simply impossible.

Adequate resistance or weight selection becomes not just important, but vital to triggering the muscle growth process. And this is where the trouble can start if your biomechanics are incorrect. This is a huge subject that gets very little attention outside of the Olympic training camps. I even see professional athletes training in videos, and a significant portion of their exercise form sucks. It is incorrect. That is where injuries start to rear their heads because of the higher loads of resistance needed to trigger muscle growth.

The rep ranges for virtually all resistance exercise movements that are being performed for hypertrophy and strength gains should be between 6 and 15. This does not mean there aren't any benefits to higher or even lower ranges (powerlifters will do lower reps, i.e., 1–4 reps). There is certainly a place for higher rep ranges, like when rehabbing an injury or post-surgery modalities. But when it comes to the muscle gains we are looking for in general, there is an optimal rep range that triggers greater hypertrophy. I cringe when I see people in the gym lifting 3-pound weights for 35 reps thinking they are "working out" for hypertrophy. That is a total delusion. And the trainers sit there and say nothing. Huh? Then they wonder why nothing has changed after years and years of "working out." The insanity of this is one of the many reasons America is growing sicker and weaker every year. There simply is not enough stimulus (weight) with a 3-pound dumbbell to cause a reaction (an adaptive response that signals the muscle to grow in size).

Training Intensity and Rep Ranges

1. Strength and Endurance:

   Reps: 15–25
   Intensity: ≤ 67% of 1-rep max (1-RM)
   Energy system: ATP-PC and Lactic

   Focuses on maintaining muscle force over time, ideal for endurance activities.

2. Hypertrophy (Muscle Growth):

   Reps: 6–15
   Intensity: 67%–85% of 1-RM
   Energy system: ATP-PC

   Targets muscle size; training to fatigue within this range stimulates optimal muscle development. Bodybuilders are in this range.

3. Maximum Strength:

   Reps: 3–6
   Intensity: ≥ 85% of 1-RM
   Energy system: ATP-PC

   Designed to maximize force production for heavy lifting.

4. Power:

   Reps: 1–5 (e.g., 1–2 for single-rep events, 3–5 for multi-rep events)
   Intensity: 75%–90% of 1-RM
   Energy system: ATP

   Focuses on explosive force generation for dynamic movements like Olympic lifts. This is a great definition of synchronous firing of muscle fiber.

132

Key Notes:

- Fewer repetitions with higher intensity develop strength and power.

- Moderate reps and intensity promote hypertrophy (muscle growth).

- Higher repetitions at lower intensities build endurance.

- Performing exercises to fatigue within these ranges ensures the appropriate overload for physiological adaptation and muscle fiber remodeling.

Hypertrophy Is Just the Beginning Benefit

When resistance protocols are put into place the proper way, *muscle growth is the major outcome only if adequate resistance is used*, but there are so many other factors that get turned on as well. Remember— resistance training means applying force against your body that requires your muscle to counteract and resist that force by firing motor units. This can be achieved by using dumbbells, cables, rubber bands, barbells, kettlebells, body weight, etc. Here are a few other major benefits triggered by resistance training:

- Bone density increases

- Fat metabolism increases

- IL-10 growth factors (see Section 4: The Fitness Science Matters)

- Synovial fluid production (see Section 4: The Fitness Science Matters)

- Central nervous system firing (see Section 4: The Fitness Science Matters)

- Stabilizer (balance) response increases

- Joint integrity increases

- Range of motion increases

- Optimized oxygen distribution

- Mitochondrial density increases (during 16+ rep range and when combined with cardio) (see Section 4: The Fitness Science Matters)

- Capillary density increases (during 16+ rep range and when combined with cardio) (see Section 4: The Fitness Science Matters)

Muscle Fiber Type 1 and Type 2

Muscle fibers in the skeletal system come in two fundamental types, each showcasing unique contractile and metabolic profiles. This diversity in muscle fiber types contributes to a wide range of performance capabilities. The two primary types are slow-twitch (type 1) and fast-twitch (type 2) fibers. Slow-twitch fibers contract and relax at a slower pace but boast a high number of mitochondria (energy storage sites in muscle), resulting in greater oxidative aerobic capacity. Activities such as running, biking, and swimming heavily rely on slow-twitch fibers due to their endurance-oriented characteristics. These fibers are richly supplied with capillaries, facilitating oxygen and nutrient transport while removing waste products. In contrast, fast-twitch (type 2) fibers contract and relax rapidly with higher force, featuring a greater glycolytic capacity and storage for high-energy phosphates and glycogen. However, they contain fewer mitochondria and capillaries.

Slow-twitch fibers demonstrate superior endurance by resisting fatigue compared to fast-twitch fibers, which are utilized for short bursts of high-intensity activities. Activities like sprinting, explosive jumps, or rapid directional changes in sports like basketball and football heavily recruit fast-twitch fibers. Despite their quick response and power, fast-twitch fibers fatigue quickly due to lactic acid build-up from anaerobic metabolism.

Genetic predisposition determines the proportion of these fiber types in an individual, with the average person having a roughly fifty-fifty split. Elite athletes often exhibit skewed percentages of these fibers, significantly influencing their athletic performance and chosen sports. For instance, a world-class sprinter possesses a higher percentage of fast-twitch fibers (type 2), while a marathon runner has a higher proportion of slow-twitch fibers (type 1). Nonetheless, all muscle fibers can adapt to specific training stimuli, enhancing their ability to cater to various athletic demands. Aerobic training can increase the aerobic metabolic capacity of fast-twitch fibers by boosting mitochondrial density, while anaerobic training can enhance the phosphagen system in slow-twitch fibers.

The velocity of muscle contraction is determined by the force and speed of contraction. Muscle contraction force and speed are dictated by the type and quantity of muscle fibers, as well as the frequency of their activation. Slow-twitch fibers are initially activated during low-intensity exercises, and as the force requirements increase, fast-twitch fibers are sequentially recruited. This systematic mobilization of muscle fibers ensures the adaptation of contraction patterns to meet specific tension, speed, and metabolic needs.

The controlled recruitment patterns of muscle fibers play a pivotal role in determining success in various athletic activities. Weightlifters and sprinters can recruit a high number of both fast-twitch and slow-twitch fibers simultaneously, generating rapid and substantial force. In contrast, endurance athletes exhibit a sequential or asynchronous recruitment pattern, relying heavily on slow oxidative fibers during prolonged activities. This recruitment pattern allows for mini-recovery periods during the activity, a luxury not available to fast-twitch fibers.

Adaptation is a multifaceted process through which muscles respond to exercise stimuli, leading to a wide range of physiological and metabolic changes. The specificity principle underlines that the gains achieved through training are specific to the activity, volume, and intensity of the exercise performed. Therefore, training programs need to align with a person's desired outcome, whether it's muscle growth or performance gains. Different training protocols result in distinct metabolic and physiological adaptations. For instance, endurance athletes enhance their aerobic power and endurance, exhibiting adaptations in both the cardiovascular and skeletal muscle systems. Cardiovascular adaptations involve an increase in heart weight, left ventricular chamber size, blood volume, and capillary density, all contributing to improved blood and oxygen flow during exercise.

Resistance or weight training, on the other hand, triggers physiological and neurological adaptations. In the initial stages, strength gains primarily stem from improvements in the central nervous system, proprioception, motor unit recruitment, and connective tissue strength. Subsequently, as connective tissue adapts and strengthens, a noticeable muscle mass increase occurs, requiring more tension to trigger the sensors in tendons. This coordinated adaptation of muscle and connective tissue contributes to increased strength and larger muscles. Understanding these intricate adaptations is crucial for tailoring effective training programs to achieve specific fitness goals. This is the exact reason why adequate resistance and the speed of the exercise movement are vitally important to building muscle on the human frame. Remember, more muscle equals a larger engine in your body, which in turn means more calories (fuel/fat) burned every second of the day! This is the way to turn your metabolic engines on and start to lose that stubborn fat.

The Science of Synchronous Versus Asynchronous Firing

In muscle physiology, synchronous and asynchronous firing refer to the coordination, timing, and amount of muscle fiber contractions during muscle activation. These firing patterns play a crucial role in muscle hypertrophy and are particularly significant for the aging population seeking to maintain or increase muscle mass.

1. **Synchronous Firing:** Synchronous firing occurs when a group of muscle fibers within a muscle contract simultaneously, generating a powerful and coordinated force. This synchronized contraction is essential for lifting heavy weights and performing

intense exercises. During synchronous firing, motor units, which are nerve-muscle fiber units, receive signals from the nervous system simultaneously, causing the muscle fibers they innervate to contract in unison. This coordinated contraction enables efficient force production and allows for lifting heavier loads during strength training exercises.

Example: When lifting a heavy barbell during a bench press, multiple motor units in the pectoral muscles contract synchronously to generate the force required to lift the weight.

2. **Asynchronous Firing:** In contrast, asynchronous firing involves motor units contracting in a staggered or alternating manner. This firing pattern is more sustainable for endurance-type activities or activities that require a more sustained muscle contraction without fatigue. Asynchronous firing helps in maintaining muscle function during prolonged or repetitive movements and is crucial for activities like long-distance running or maintaining posture.

Example: During a sustained plank exercise, different motor units in the core muscles fire asynchronously to maintain the position and support the body weight.

3. **Importance for Hypertrophy and the Aging Population:**

a. **Hypertrophy:** Synchronous firing is particularly important for muscle hypertrophy, which refers to the increase in muscle size. When muscle fibers contract synchronously under substantial resistance (e.g., weightlifting using appropriate weights), it leads to microtears in those fibers. The body then repairs these tears during the recovery process, resulting in muscle growth and increased muscle mass. Using adequate resistance ensures that synchronous firing occurs optimally, promoting hypertrophy.

b. **Aging and Muscle Loss:** As individuals age, there is a natural decline in muscle mass and strength known as sarcopenia, which we touched on earlier. This loss of muscle mass can lead to decreased mobility, frailty, and an increased risk of falls and fractures in the elderly. Incorporating resistance training with an emphasis on synchronous firing into the exercise routine is crucial for aging individuals. It helps counteract muscle loss by stimulating muscle fibers to contract synchronously against resistance, promoting muscle growth, strength, and overall functional ability.

c. **Optimizing Synchronous Firing in Resistance Training:** Using enough resistance during resistance training sessions is pivotal to triggering greater synchronous firing in muscle fibers. This, in turn, maximizes muscle activation and promotes hypertrophy. The aging population should be guided to use appropriate resistance levels in their exercises to ensure optimal synchronous firing and gain the benefits of increased muscle mass and strength.

Synchronous firing patterns, where a higher percentage of muscle fibers contract together (slow-twitch type 1 fibers along with fast-twitch type 2 fibers), is vital for generating significant force during exercises, promoting muscle hypertrophy. For the aging population combating muscle loss, optimizing synchronous firing through resistance training is crucial to maintain or increase muscle mass, enhance strength, and improve overall quality of life. I dive in with a little more detail and examples of synchronous patterns in section 4, "The Fitness Science Matters."

Bioenergetics

Bioenergetics is the study of energy types and usage through living systems, particularly focusing on the conversion of energy from food into a form usable by cells, such as adenosine triphosphate (ATP). Understanding the basics of bioenergetics is crucial in comprehending the physiological processes that enable organisms to perform various activities, from simple cellular functions to complex physical tasks like athletic performance.

The process of bioenergetics involves several phases, each utilizing different energy systems to generate ATP:

ATP-PC (Phosphagen) System: This system provides immediate energy for short bursts of high-intensity activities, such as sprinting or weightlifting. It relies on stored ATP and phosphocreatine (PC) reserves in the muscle cells. When ATP is broken down into adenosine diphosphate (ADP) and inorganic phosphate (Pi), the energy released helps fuel muscle contraction. The ATP-PC system is anaerobic, meaning it does not require oxygen. However, it is limited in its capacity and can only sustain activity for a short duration, typically 10–15 seconds.

Lactic Acid (Glycolytic) System: When the ATP-PC system is depleted, the body switches to the glycolytic system, which generates energy through the breakdown of glucose. This system can operate anaerobically or aerobically but is primarily anaerobic during high-intensity activities. Glucose is converted into pyruvate through glycolysis, producing ATP in the process. Under anaerobic conditions or when oxygen availability is limited, pyruvate is converted into lactate, leading to the accumulation of lactic acid in the muscles. The lactic acid system provides energy for activities lasting from about 30 seconds to 2 minutes, making it essential for events like 400-meter sprints or intense weightlifting.

Anaerobic (Glycolytic) System: This system is an extension of the lactic acid system and continues to provide energy through glycolysis, but without the accumulation of lactate. Instead, pyruvate is converted into other by-products such as acetyl-CoA, which can enter the aerobic energy system for further ATP production. The anaerobic system is still predominantly utilized during high-intensity activities lasting up to two minutes, but it becomes increasingly important as the duration of the activity extends beyond the capabilities of the ATP-PC and lactic acid systems.

Aerobic (Oxidative) System: The aerobic system is the most efficient energy system, utilizing oxygen to produce ATP through the breakdown of carbohydrates, fats, and proteins. Aerobic metabolism occurs in the mitochondria and is capable of sustaining prolonged, low- to moderate-intensity activities, such as distance running or cycling. Carbohydrates are broken down into pyruvate, which enters the citric acid cycle (Krebs cycle) and electron transport chain to generate ATP.

Beta-Oxidation: Aerobic activity past three minutes involves the use of fats (or lipids) that undergo oxidation to produce acetyl-CoA, which also enters the citric acid cycle. This aerobic system provides the majority of the energy for endurance activities lasting more than a few minutes and is crucial for events like marathons or long-distance cycling races.

To illustrate the utilization of these energy systems, let's compare a sprinter and a marathon runner:

Sprinter, Shot Put, Bodybuilder: During a sprint, a sprinter primarily relies on the ATP-PC system and the lactic acid system. The short, intense nature of the sprint places high demands on immediate energy sources, making the ATP-PC system essential for the initial explosive bursts. As the sprint progresses, the glycolytic system becomes increasingly important, providing energy through the breakdown of glucose to sustain muscle contraction. However, the sprint is too short for significant aerobic metabolism to occur.

Marathon Runner: In contrast, a marathon runner primarily utilizes the aerobic system. The long duration of the marathon requires a sustained, steady supply of energy, which is efficiently provided by aerobic metabolism. Fats are the predominant fuel source during endurance activities, with carbohydrates serving as a secondary fuel. The marathon runner's aerobic capacity allows for the continuous production of ATP through oxidative phosphorylation, enabling them to maintain pace over the extended distance.

The understanding of bioenergetics and the different energy systems is essential for optimizing athletic performance across various activities, from short bursts of high-intensity effort to prolonged endurance events. Each energy system plays a specific role in meeting the energy demands of different types of physical exertion, with the balance between them varying depending on the duration and intensity of the activity.

Biomechanics and Understanding GTOs Are Vital

As stated earlier, biomechanics is the technical term for exercise form. Nothing could be more important than this. Sorry to say, but proper biomechanics is virtually nonexistent at every gym I have ever been to. Probably 95% of all the trainers I have ever watched—which number in the hundreds—are unaware of how to properly explain them, let alone teach them properly. It is truly awful. I don't blame them entirely. I know a lot of trainers and most of them are awesome people trying to make a difference, but they just don't have the appropriate knowledge. I blame the $80 billion fitness industry that promotes monthly dues and group training-wrecks instead of proper fitness science and protocols, which all rest on a few major vital principles, one being proper biomechanics.

Exercise form is so vital. It's what prevents injuries, maximizes muscle motor unit recruitment, and increases hypertrophy, which is directly required to achieve any success with fitness.

One of the most important lessons to understand is that bad or improper exercise form leads to Golgi tendon organ (GTO) triggering by excessive torque in the connective (joint) tissue, thus leading to less muscle motor unit recruitment during the exercise. This is the opposite of what you're trying to accomplish in a workout. This leads to an exponential loss of muscle gains (hypertrophy) and a higher probability of injuries. This is why biomechanics are crucial to your gains and success and is one of our biggest educational components with our clients. It is barely talked about inside the gym because nobody understands it, has ever heard about it, or can intelligently explain the importance of this process.

GTO'S – A VITAL PIECE OF FITNESS SCIENCE

This is one of the most important pieces of science for achieving your success when it comes to maximizing muscle gain and avoiding injuries in The FITNESS QUADRANT system—particularly the resistance training quadrant.

Once you understand this, you'll take a gigantic leap forward to success. This is a crucial part of our onboarding process, as it sets the stage for all our clients to have massive success and training longevity in their journey of living strong and most of all avoiding unnecessary injuries.

The Golgi tendon organs (GTOs) are specialized proprioceptors located within the tendons near the muscle-tendon junction. These sensory receptors play a crucial role in regulating muscle tension and preventing excessive force during muscle contractions, particularly in the context of weight training or any activity that demands physical exertion.

The GTOs function as a feedback mechanism, constantly monitoring changes in muscle tension. When a muscle contracts, the attached tendon is stretched, activating the GTOs. This activation initiates a sensory signal sent to the central nervous system, specifically to the spinal cord, where it synapses with motor neurons.

Poor biomechanics (exercise form) means that the joint is not at the correct angle, *which multiplies the tension on the connective tissue*, thus triggering GTOs that shut down the muscle motor firing. This means your intended exercise is not overloading the muscle, it is overloading the connective tissue. This means inadequate tension gets put through the muscle resulting in extremely low gains through adaptive response. There simply is not enough stimulus in the muscle to trigger hypertrophy. Bottom line? A gigantic waste of time that nets zero results you are looking for.

When the GTOs detect high levels of tension in the muscle-tendon complex, signaling that the muscle is generating a force near its maximum capability, they trigger an inhibitory reflex. This reflex results in a reduction of motor neuron activity, essentially shutting down or inhibiting further muscle recruitment. This mechanism is known as autogenic inhibition.

The purpose of this inhibition is to prevent muscle damage or excessive force that could lead to injury. For instance, if you're weightlifting and attempting to lift a weight that is too heavy for your muscle or connective tissue due to improper biomechanics to handle, the GTOs will sense the excessive tension and inhibit further force generation. This process is designed to protect the muscle from potential tears or other injuries that might occur if force were to continue to be applied.

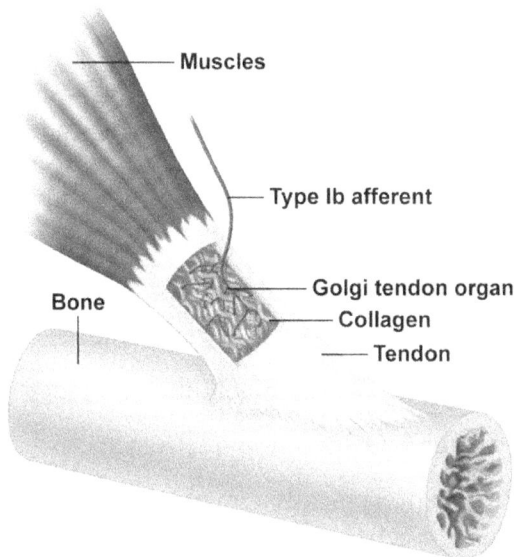

© 2011 Pearson Education. Inc

Conversely, when the GTOs detect a decrease in tension, such as during stretching or relaxation of the muscle, they reduce their inhibitory effect. This allows for a controlled contraction and prevents unnecessary inhibition of muscle activity.

Understanding the function of GTOs is crucial for athletes, trainers, and individuals engaged in weight training. It underscores the importance of proper form, posture, and alignment during exercises to optimize muscle engagement while minimizing the risk of injury. By maintaining correct biomechanics (exercise form), joint angles, and positioning from *proper* technique, individuals can work with their GTOs to achieve efficient muscle recruitment and maximize the benefits of their training regimen.

Why would you "train like an animal" to try to "look good" and just "work through the pain" when in reality your joints and body are being torn to shreds and in constant pain? Huh? This is the lowest form of fitness on the planet. This mentality is a black eye and a problem for the entire fitness industry, but few address it because only a few realize it.

Concentric Versus Eccentric Muscle Firing Phases: Key Differences

Muscle movement during exercise is classified into concentric and eccentric phases, each with unique characteristics and roles in strength development and hypertrophy.

Concentric Phase (Muscle Shortening)

- **Definition:** The phase where the muscle actively contracts and shortens, generating force to move a load.

- **Example:** Lifting the dumbbell during a bicep curl.

- **Primary Focus:** Overcoming resistance.

- **Load-Bearing:** Typically involves lower force output, as muscles are mechanically less capable of handling as much weight during concentric contractions.

Eccentric Phase (Muscle Lengthening)

- **Definition:** The phase where the muscle lengthens under tension, controlling the descent or resisting the force of gravity.

- **Example:** Lowering the dumbbell during a bicep curl.

- **Primary Focus:** Resisting or decelerating the load.

- **Load-Bearing:** During this phase, muscles can handle 120%–160% more load compared to during the concentric phase, making eccentric contractions inherently stronger.

- **Muscle Damage:** Most microscopic muscle damage occurs during the eccentric phase due to the higher force demands and mechanical strain. This damage triggers the repair process essential for hypertrophy.

Hypertrophy and Eccentric Loading

- **Eccentric Importance:** The controlled elongation of muscles under high tension is where the majority of structural stress occurs. This stress creates microscopic tears in the muscle fibers, which the body repairs during recovery (nutrition!), leading to stronger and larger muscles.

- **Training Applications:**
  - Incorporating eccentric-focused exercises (e.g., slow negatives) can maximize hypertrophy potential.
  - Exercises designed to emphasize the eccentric phase often lead to greater muscle soreness (delayed onset muscle soreness, or DOMS) due to the increased damage.

By understanding and leveraging the differences between these phases, individuals can optimize their training for strength and muscle growth. Emphasizing controlled eccentric movements can significantly enhance hypertrophic adaptations.

N = NUTRITION
(top right quadrant)

You cannot out-exercise poor nutrition.

This is where proper nutrients repair and grow muscle and also fuel your body and brain. Nutrition is something you need to get right if you're going to tap into the power and success of living in growth mode by triggering anabolic responses. It is very easy to slip into decay with food because it is very easy and convenient to find toxic food—it's everywhere. It takes work and planning to eat quality nutritious food—in the proper amounts. Resistance training workouts generally take less than an hour if you're doing them properly, and that's only 2 to 4 days per week. But food is a 16-hour battle (you're sleeping for 7 to 8 hours), 7 days a week! You have to stay committed enough to stay in a zone. This is why nutrition is harder than working out. However, after a while, when you've learned how to eat properly, it becomes automatic, and you don't even think about it because it has become a lifestyle. And that's where you want to get to.

Although, with a little knowledge and commitment, the components of a healthy diet are easy to understand and not that difficult to practice; unfortunately, most people don't. The delusion of weight loss and trying to out-exercise poor nutrition habits is a prevailing condition in society. Many people engage in fitness and treat it as an *offset* to a toxic lifestyle—inadequate nutrition, excessive alcohol, poor eating habits, and toxic food choices. It's a quick nosedive if you're not serious about it. Superior fitness is a combination of many components, with the bedrock being accurate science-driven resistance training, sound nutrition, and cardiovascular bouts. No pills, no fad diets, and please, no fad workout routines—stop the insanity. Avoid processed sugars, trans fats, and all processed foods. These three things are very stealthy and will eventually kill you. Garbage Instagram and YouTube influencer workout routines will never make up for poor nutrition. Period. If you do not get resistance training and great nutrition right, you will fail to capture the true benefits of fitness, wellness, and longevity. If you're going to do it, *do it right*. Stop the fake fitness pipedream.

Nutrition is a hot topic for most people. There is so much information out there. Some of it is accurate. However, a very large portion of it is completely false and misleading, thanks to the multibillion-dollar companies and "weight loss" cronies making money off selling you psychological hope of losing weight. It's infuriating to me because I see lots and lots of great people struggling with this every day.

A basic understanding of nutrition goes a long way. Nutrition is like the two-by-fours and nails for repairing and fueling your body—complete proteins for building/repairing muscle tissue and carbohydrates and fats for fueling your body's energy needs. Your body also needs adequate nutrients in the form of minerals and vitamins, and phytonutrients from fruits and veggies. Whole or complete proteins—ones that contain the nine essential amino acids that are only supplied through dietary intake—help in remodeling muscle proteins in the muscle or fasciculi. In other words, they add actin and myosin filaments, which are comprised of proteins—more muscle. Great fitness routines are nullified without good nutrition to support the energy and repair requirements from the workouts. Conversely, good nutrition alone will not add muscle to your body. Adequate resistance modalities are the stimulus required for muscle growth, protein repairs the damage.

Before we get into the details of proper nutrition, here are some basic pointers that are not so basic when you internalize them.

Always select whole foods. Remember, the closer to the earth your food sources are, the better. The more processed and refined or "convenient" the foods, the more hands have touched your food, the more fake and chemical laced the food is and the higher and more damaging the calories are. And worse, these are "empty" calories meaning they have very low nutritional value to you when compared to earth foods. Stay away from it at all costs. This is a gigantic issue. Choose wisely. Your life depends on it. Here is an example:

Calorie Comparison: Fast Food vs Whole Food

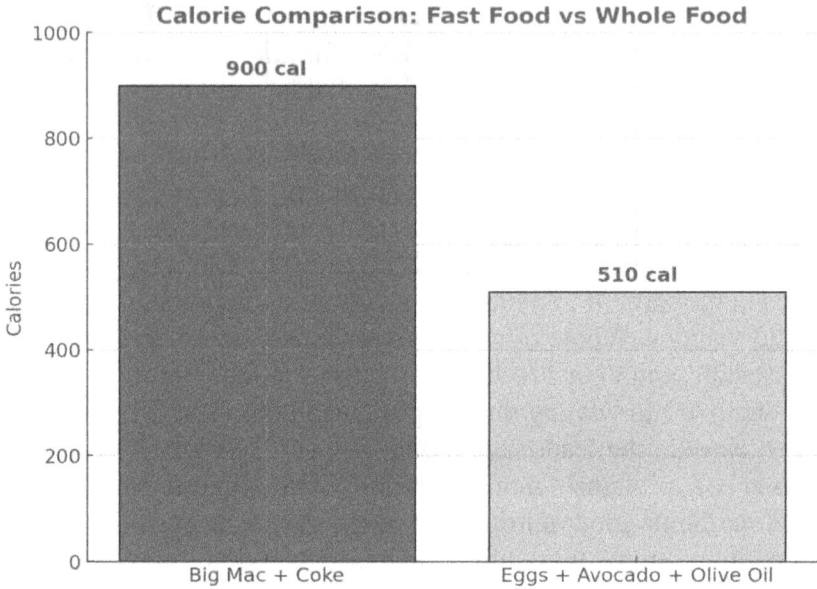

Processed Fast Food Meal

- Big Mac: ~590 calories
- Large Coke: ~310 calories
- Total: ~900 calories

Mostly refined carbs, added sugars, unhealthy fats, and low nutrient density.

Whole food Meal

- 5 whole eggs: ~350 calories
- ½ avocado: ~120 calories
- 1 tsp olive oil: ~40 calories
- Total: ~510 calories

High in protein, healthy fats, vitamins, and minerals. Nutrient-dense and keeps you fuller longer.

The Takeaway: The highly processed fast-food option is nearly 400 more calories with little nutrition, while the whole food option gives you superior protein, healthy fats, and micronutrients—fueling your body rather than spiking insulin and storing fat.

To start, establish a consistent baseline. Eat three main meals per day. The average non-workout person should consume approximately 1,600 to 2,200 calories per day. Obviously, this is a blanket range not intended to be specific. It's good place to start for most people. It's what comprises these caloric values that matters, meaning, are you eating empty calories or nutrient dense calories? Divide these calories by three meals and it translates into about 550 to 750 calories per meal. A great starting ratio of proteins/carbs/fats is a 40/30/30 split. This simply means out of the calories you are consuming, allocate 40% to protein and 30% to each carbs and good fats. Protein and carbs have 4 calories per gram and fats have 9 calories per gram. Below is the basic math on how you determine how much protein/carbs/fats to consume on a 1,600 total daily calorie nutrition plan with a 40/30/30 macro split. This is a good basic start and how to understand ratios of macros consumed on a daily basis. It gets more detailed and complex from here.

1,600 calories x 40% (pro) = 640 protein calories
or 640/4 = 160 grams of protein daily

1,600 calories x 30% (carbs) = 480 carb calories
or 480/4 = 120 grams of carbs daily

1,600 calories x 30% (fats) = 480 fat calories
or 480/9 = 53 grams of fats daily

Determine the amount of protein you need daily, and there are many different ways to do this, depending on the person, their goals, and the timeline. For general purposes, here is an easy formula to follow for the non-competitive individual who has a much lower protein turnover rate (protein requirement) compared to an active athlete or fitness enthusiast.

Body Weight x 70% = Protein Intake in Grams

Example: 215 lb. male X 70% = 150.5 grams
of whole proteins daily or 50 grams/meal

Again, this is for a non-athlete and someone who doesn't work out, other than maybe walking or light sporting such as golf on the weekend. (The % ratio would be more like 90%+ for the active athlete and even higher for a competitive bodybuilder, closer to 125%). The above example could start you out, then you tweak from there.

The average sedentary person can greatly benefit from getting a proper amount of whole proteins. If this person started working out on a regular basis, their daily need for protein would increase on a sliding scale depending on the type, volume, and intensity of the workouts. Protein would then scale as a percentage of the 150 grams—i.e., add 10% to your total daily proteins for every day you train. If you train three days per week, add 30% to your total daily protein intake to make up for the added protein turnover from training. A good legitimate athletic trainer who also understands nutrition (and has lots of experience) can help you get detailed on this. They provide invaluable customized information to help you reach your goals.

Eat from a select menu of high-quality proteins, carbs, and fats that are as close as possible to the source, i.e., a farm or credible whole food store for produce and protein.

Eat lots of vegetables and whole fruits with your protein.

I do not get any of my main food from the grocery store. I buy from local farms or high-end small purveyors that buy directly from truly organic farms.

Protein: Farm eggs, grass-fed red meat (from a local farm), bison, venison, wild salmon, chicken, turkey, tuna, haddock, swordfish, beef liver, ocean-caught shrimp and scallops, raw milk, cottage cheese, Greek yogurt, grass-fed whey protein powder.

Carbs – complex: Egg bagel, rice, sweet and white potatoes, imported or homemade pasta, sourdough bread from local bakery.

Carbs – simple: Bananas, blueberries, sumo oranges, apples, kiwis, broccoli, spinach, asparagus, kale, mushrooms, garden tomatoes, cucumbers, zucchini, garlic, onions, local honey, local maple syrup.

Fats: Avocados, salmon, red meat, dairy, butter, olive oil (only high quality such as Ariston), coconut oil, avocado oil, grass-fed ghee, peanut butter, almond butter.

Hydration: I drink only filtered water that I mineralize with ocean minerals (supplements section), or legitimate bottled water (glass bottles) that has trace minerals and lithium in it, and lots of coconut water that I add sea salt to. This is 95% of my fluid intake.

Here is a friendly reminder of what we discussed about toxic foods and that it should be your #1 priority to cut them out of your life. Understanding the toxic foods that kill you slowly is a *major* part of nutrition acumen. You must know what foods to avoid just as much as knowing what foods to incorporate in order to trigger growth and avoid decay.

The top three foods to avoid are sugar, trans fats, and seed oils—these are either stand-alone products or in *all* processed foods. Remember, these are three of the horsemen of sickness. Avoid them like the plague. It sounds simple, but the cold hard facts say differently. Sugar and trans fats can be found in literally 95% of the mass-produced foods you'll find in every grocery store on every corner of Main Street, USA. Even "health food stores" are now filled with garbage products and garbage ingredients like seed oils and sugars that look and claim to be organic and wholesome. Whole Foods isn't as "whole" as you think. It is littered with crap foods and drinks that appear healthy and are everything but. There are over forty-eight different names for chemically made sweeteners and processed fats that are—quite interestingly—legal to use on food labels. Hmm… Can you say billions of dollars in profits for Wall Street and multinational food producers? You bet.

There are two major categories of nutrition:

1. **Macronutrients** – Protein, carbohydrates, fats
2. **Micronutrients** – Vitamins and minerals

Macronutrients

The essential components of our diet that provide energy and serve various vital functions in the body. There are three main macronutrients: carbohydrates, proteins, and fats.

Carbohydrates are the primary source of energy for the body. They are made up of sugar molecules and are found in foods like rice, pasta, potato, grains, fruits, vegetables, and legumes. Carbohydrates are broken down into glucose, which is used by the body for energy production. They also play a role in supporting brain function and providing fiber for digestive health.

Proteins are essential for muscle growth, repair, and maintenance of all other tissues in the body. They are made up of amino acids, which are often referred to as the building blocks of proteins. Proteins are found in foods like meat, poultry, fish, eggs, dairy products, legumes, and nuts. They are involved in various bodily functions, including enzyme production, immune system support, and hormone regulation.

Fats are concentrated sources of energy and are crucial for cell structure, hormone production, and nutrient absorption. They are divided into categories such as saturated fats, unsaturated fats (including monounsaturated and polyunsaturated fats), and trans fats. Sources of healthy fats include avocados, nuts, seeds, olive oil, and fatty fish. While fats are often associated with weight gain, they are necessary and good for overall health when consumed in moderation.

Basic Functions of Each Macronutrient

Carbohydrates: Rice, pasta, potato, bread/(simple) carbs, fruits, and veggies

Primary source of energy

Support brain function

Provide dietary fiber for digestive health

Proteins (*Whole): Eggs, red meat, chicken, turkey, dairy, fish, organ meat

Essential for all tissue growth, muscle hypertrophy, repair, and maintenance

Involved in enzyme production

Support immune function

Regulate hormone activity

*Nine Essential Amino Acids Only Found in Whole Proteins:

Histidine
Isoleucine
Leucine
Lysine
Methionine

Phenylalanine
Threonine
Tryptophan
Valine

Fats (good fats): Avocado, butter, olive oil, fish, meats, nuts, whole dairy

Concentrated source of energy

Essential for cell structure and function

Aid in hormone production and regulation

Facilitate the absorption of fat-soluble vitamins

Micronutrients

Essential vitamins and minerals required by the body in small quantities for various physiological functions. Unlike macronutrients, which mainly provide energy and tissue repair, micronutrients play other critical roles in metabolism, immune function, growth, and overall health. They are primarily obtained through a balanced diet, although supplements may be necessary in cases of deficiency or for high performance activities like sports.

Micronutrients are found in a wide range of foods, including fruits, vegetables, whole grains, nuts, seeds, dairy products, meats, and seafood. Each vitamin and mineral comes from specific food sources, and consuming a diverse array of nutrient-rich foods ensures adequate intake of micronutrients.

Basic Functions of Micronutrients

Vitamin A: Supports vision, immune function, and skin health.

Vitamin B Complex: Includes several vitamins (B1, B2, B3, B5, B6, B7, B9, B12) involved in energy metabolism, nervous system function, red blood cell formation, and DNA synthesis.

Vitamin C: Acts as an antioxidant, supports immune function, collagen synthesis, and enhances iron absorption.

Vitamin D: Essential for bone health, calcium absorption, immune function, and cell growth regulation.

Vitamin E: Functions as an antioxidant, protects cells from damage, and supports immune function.

Vitamin K: Important for blood clotting, bone metabolism, and heart health.

Calcium: Vital for bone and teeth health, muscle function, nerve transmission, and blood clotting.

Iron: Essential for oxygen transport, energy production, and immune function.

Magnesium: Supports muscle and nerve function, bone health, energy metabolism, and protein synthesis.

Zinc: Plays a role in immune function, wound healing, DNA synthesis, and cell division.

Selenium: Acts as an antioxidant, supports thyroid function, and plays a role in immune response.

Iodine: Essential for thyroid hormone production, which regulates metabolism and growth.

Potassium: Important for fluid balance, nerve transmission, muscle contraction, and heart function.

Sodium: Regulates fluid balance, nerve function, and muscle contraction.

Micronutrients are indispensable for overall health and well-being, despite being required only in small amounts. Consuming a varied and balanced diet rich in fruits, vegetables, whole grains, lean proteins, and dairy products ensures adequate intake of the essential vitamins and minerals necessary for optimal physiological function.

My Personal Daily Food Choices

This is 99% of my substrate intake 24/7/365

PROTEIN (whole)	CARBOHYDRATES	FATS
Eggs	Egg/sourdough bagel (morning)	Olive oil (Ariston brand)
All red meats	Rice (up to lunch only)	
Fish (salmon, whitefish, tuna)	Pasta (up to lunch only)	
Whey protein (shake)	Sweet or regular potato (up to lunch only)	
Chicken	*Whole fruits – lots every meal	
Turkey	**Veggies – lots every meal	Peanut butter
Beef liver	Avocados	Almond butter
Cottage cheese	Local honey (served on my protein)	Avocados
Greek yogurt		Ghee
Milk, raw		Beef tallow

FRUITS: Bananas, blueberries (tons), oranges, pears, apples, strawberries, kiwis, pineapple, peaches, grapes

****VEGGIES:** Broccoli, kale, beets, cucumbers, asparagus, onions, garlic, carrots, arugula, red cabbage, spinach, fresh whole leaf basil.

I personally favor fruits more than veggies in my daily nutrition, probably a 60/40 ratio. I eat quite a bit of both along with my protein of choice. They taste better and are just easier to use in my shakes (bananas, blueberries) and I actually grill pineapple and peaches often along with onions and asparagus and red cabbage. Simple, lots of fiber and delicious with olive oil salt and pepper!

When it comes to vegetables, there is a current debate about oxalates and lectins in veggies. Oxalates and lectins are naturally occurring compounds found in many plant foods, especially leafy greens like spinach, beans, and kale. Oxalates can bind to minerals like calcium and iron, making them harder for the body to absorb, and in high amounts may contribute to kidney stone formation in susceptible people. Lectins, found in beans, legumes, and some vegetables, are proteins that can interfere with nutrient absorption and may cause digestive irritation in sensitive individuals if eaten in excess or undercooked. I personally do not eat beans often. It is a very poor choice for protein compared to eggs, red meat, turkey, salmon, raw milk etc. and I find it is hard to digest easily. I like to enjoy my food and not feel like I am having an additional workout just to digest it.

That said, vegetables also provide *tremendous benefits*: fiber for gut health, vitamins for immunity, minerals for energy and bone strength, and antioxidants that protect against disease. The key is *balance*— eating a variety of vegetables, properly preparing foods (e.g., cooking beans to reduce lectins), and not overloading on any single high-oxalate food like spinach. In moderation, vegetables remain one of the most powerful foundations for long-term health and vitality.

Adequate protein intake (and type) is a requirement for muscle maintenance/growth (you should have your daily protein amount measured in grams per ounce then broken down into grams per meal).

I consume very low or zero complex carbs (rice, pasta, potatoes, bread) after lunch—especially at dinner. My dinner (around 5:30 p.m.) consists of whole proteins, fruits, and veggies only.

There is such a wide range of factors that determine what food (and how many calories) you should be consuming daily. I give a basic breakdown of this and a basic workout program (resistance and cardio) at the end of this section. It will hopefully help give you a target to start from. Remember, when we work with our clients, we are constantly modifying all these modalities because our clients are constantly changing as they get more and more fit. You can always reach out to us if you're ever interested in working with one of our various programs. Our links are in the back of the book.

Now, let's talk about your drinking water.

WATER: A Major Toxicity Problem for Many

Get your water source right. As we covered in "Your Toxic World" in Section 2, if you're drinking from a public water system, or a majority of the plastic bottled water on the market, you're most likely consuming toxins and microplastics and you're literally sacrificing your health and longevity along with nullifying your efforts in your fitness training. You have to get your water right if you want to stay away from potentially very bad health outcomes. You have to source chemical-free pure spring water that is loaded with natural minerals and has zero of the fluoride and other additives found in the public water supply. It is a must. Or, if you're economically able, invest in a high-quality reverse osmosis system for your house or apartment. It is worth every dime.

> **Fluoride:** A dangerous neurotoxin in your water supplies. It's unfortunately touted for its "benefits" in preventing tooth decay and is often added to drinking water, toothpaste, and other dental hygiene products. However, our constant exposure to fluoride, especially through water fluoridation and certain dental products, has raised concerns due to its neurotoxic effects in humans.

> **Water Fluoridation:** Public health organizations promote water fluoridation to prevent tooth decay. However, excessive levels of fluoride in drinking water, often due to fluoridation, poses serious health risks. The acceptable level of fluoride in drinking water

varies by country, but exceeding these levels can lead to overexposure. Fluoride is a neurotoxin and is absolutely not needed in any excessive amount in your body.

Neurotoxicity: Numerous studies have raised concerns about the neurotoxic effects of fluoride. *Minerals for the Genetic Code* by Charles Waters discusses the impact of excessive fluoride on the nervous system, highlighting that it can potentially lead to cognitive impairments, especially in children.

Dental Fluorosis: Excessive fluoride exposure during tooth development in childhood can lead to dental fluorosis, a cosmetic issue affecting tooth enamel. Severe fluorosis can result in brown discoloration and pitting of the teeth.

Skeletal Fluorosis: Prolonged exposure to high levels of fluoride can lead to skeletal fluorosis, a condition affecting bones and joints. It causes pain, limited mobility, and skeletal deformities.

Thyroid Dysfunction: Some studies suggest that excessive fluoride intake interferes with thyroid function and can potentially lead to hypothyroidism.

Endocrine Disruption: Fluoride disrupts the endocrine system, affecting hormone regulation and leading to various health issues.

Cancer Risk: While research on this link is ongoing, some studies have explored potential connections between long-term exposure to fluoride and an increased risk of osteosarcoma, a type of bone cancer.

Developmental Disorders: High fluoride exposure during early development years may have detrimental effects on cognitive function, behavior, and IQ.

Protein Quality Rankings

It is important to understand the biological value (BV) in choosing complete proteins. A protein source with a BV of 100 implies that all the nitrogen absorbed is retained by the body, indicating optimal protein utilization. Different protein sources exhibit varying BVs, reflecting their amino acid profiles and digestibility. Proteins derived from animal sources have higher BVs compared to plant-based proteins due to their more complete amino acid profiles.

Eggs are often considered the gold standard for protein quality, boasting a BV of approximately 100. The amino acid composition of egg protein closely matches the body's needs, making it an excellent source for muscle protein synthesis and overall growth.

Whey protein, especially in the form of whey protein isolate, is renowned for its high BV. Whey protein isolate undergoes additional processing to remove most of the fats and lactose from the whey, resulting in a protein source with a BV exceeding 100. The rapid digestion and absorption of whey protein make it a preferred choice for athletes looking to support muscle building and recovery. It helps support protein synthesis and repair damaged muscle tissues after intense workouts.

The efficiency of whey protein isolate in delivering essential amino acids to muscles quickly has led to its widespread use in sports nutrition. Athletes often consume whey protein isolate as part of their post-workout regimen to capitalize on the anabolic window when the body is primed for nutrient uptake.

Red meat, such as beef, also provides a substantial BV, typically ranging from 75 to 90. While not as high as eggs or whey protein isolate, red meat remains a valuable source of complete protein, rich in essential amino acids and vital nutrients.

Branched-Chain Amino Acids (BCAAs) are a group of essential amino acids that are vital for various physiological functions in the body. The three amino acids included in the BCAA category are:

1. Leucine
2. Isoleucine
3. Valine

Unlike other amino acids, BCAAs are unique in that they are metabolized in the muscle tissue rather than the liver, making them readily available for energy production and protein synthesis.

BV measures how efficiently the body can absorb and utilize a protein source for muscle repair, growth, and overall function. The higher the BV number, the more readily the body can use the amino acids in that protein for muscle protein synthesis. Complete proteins—those containing all nine essential amino acids—are particularly important for fitness and muscle building. Selecting high-BV proteins ensures maximum recovery, muscle retention, and overall performance. Notice that plant proteins do not even make the top fifteen list when compared to animal proteins. They are a very poor choice for muscle maintenance and repair/building.

Top Twenty Whole Proteins by BV for Muscle Building

1. **Whey Protein Isolate** – BV: 104–159 (fast digestion, optimal for recovery)
2. **Whole Egg** – BV: 100 (gold standard for natural protein)
3. **Egg White** – BV: 88 (high in leucine, excellent for lean muscle growth)
4. **Milk Protein (Casein + Whey)** – BV: 91 (supports sustained muscle repair)
5. **Beef (Lean Cuts)** – BV: 80 (rich in iron and B vitamins for strength)

6. **Chicken Breast** – BV: 79 (lean, high-protein muscle-building staple)

7. **Fish (Salmon, Tuna, Cod)** – BV: 76–83 (packed with omega-3s for recovery)

8. **Turkey Breast** – BV: 79 (low-fat, high-protein source for lean gains)

9. **Greek Yogurt** – BV: 84 (casein-rich for prolonged muscle recovery)

10. **Cottage Cheese** – BV: 81 (slow-digesting casein for muscle preservation)

11. **Bison** – BV: 79 (lean, nutrient-dense red meat alternative)

12. **Pork (Lean Cuts like Tenderloin)** – BV: 77 (rich in BCAAs for recovery)

13. **Shrimp** – BV: 85 (low-fat, high-protein seafood option)

14. **Lamb** – BV: 76 (rich in essential amino acids and iron)

15. **Venison (Deer Meat)** – BV: 74 (lean, high-protein wild-game option)

16. **Quinoa** – BV: 73 (highest BV grain, complete plant-based protein)

17. **Cheese (Parmesan, Cheddar)** – BV: 74–85 (calcium-rich muscle-building option)

18. **Duck Meat** – BV: 70 (nutrient-dense, high-quality protein option)

19. **Tempeh** – BV: 70 (fermented soy for better digestion and muscle growth)

20. **Tofu (Soy Protein)** – BV: 64 (best plant-based complete protein option)

Choosing high-BV protein sources ensures better muscle repair, sustained energy, and optimized strength gains, making them essential for any fitness-focused diet.

Carbohydrates & Glycemic Index

The glycemic index (GI) is a ranking system that measures how quickly carbohydrate-containing foods raise blood sugar levels. It is scored on a scale from 0 to 100, with pure glucose serving as the reference point (GI = 100). As a very important rule, stick with slow carbs (0–55) and avoid fast carbs (70–100).

As you'll see the list below, foods are categorized into three levels:

- **Low GI (0–55):** Slow-digesting, gradual blood sugar release.
- **Medium GI (56–69):** Moderate blood sugar response.
- **High GI (70–100):** Rapid blood sugar spike.

Here is an outline of how the GI affects the body:

1. Energy Levels

- **Low GI Foods:** Provide sustained energy, preventing energy crashes. Ideal for long-lasting mental and physical performance.
- **High GI Foods:** Cause quick spikes in energy followed by crashes, leading to fatigue and hunger soon after consumption.

2. Insulin Secretion

- **Low GI Foods:** Promote gradual insulin release, helping maintain balanced blood sugar and reducing the risk of insulin resistance.
- **High GI Foods:** Trigger rapid insulin spikes, which can lead to increased fat storage and long-term insulin resistance.

3. Fat Storage and Weight Management

- **Low GI Foods:** Support fat loss by stabilizing blood sugar and reducing cravings.

- **High GI Foods:** Encourage fat storage due to excess insulin response, which shuttles glucose into fat cells when energy needs are met.

Glycemic Index Chart

Category	Low GI (0–55)	Medium GI (56–69)	High GI (70–100)
Grains and Breads	Quinoa (53), Whole Wheat Bread (50), Steel-Cut Oats (55)	Brown Rice (66), Sourdough Bread (62), Couscous (65)	White Bread (75), Instant Oats (79), White Rice (89)
Fruits	Cherries (22), Apples (36), Grapefruit (25)	Pineapple (66), Mango (60)	Watermelon (76), Dates (103)
Vegetables	Broccoli (10), Spinach (15), Carrots (39)	Sweet Corn (60), Beetroot (64)	White Potatoes (85), Pumpkin (75)
Dairy	Greek Yogurt (35), Whole Milk (39)	Ice Cream (61)	Skimmed Milk (70)
Legumes	Lentils (32), Chickpeas (28), Black Beans (30)	Kidney Beans (52), Baked Beans (55)	
Processed Snacks	Dark Chocolate (40), Nuts (15)	Popcorn (65), Granola Bar (59)	Potato Chips (75), Doughnuts (76), Sugary Cereals (82)

Key Takeaways

- **Low GI foods** support steady energy, reduce insulin spikes, and minimize fat storage.

- **High GI foods** lead to blood sugar crashes, excess insulin secretion, and increased fat accumulation if consumed excessively.

- **Balanced meals with protein, fiber, and healthy fats** help mitigate the glycemic impact of high GI foods.

By prioritizing low GI whole foods, you can optimize energy levels, improve metabolic health, and manage body composition effectively.

The Third Major Component of Nutrition

After you grasp the basics of macros and micros, the third major component of great nutrition is a repetition of what I discussed earlier in this chapter—things to avoid. Most of the food that's readily available at your local grocery store and restaurants is toxic and mass produced. It's toxic because it contains the four toxic additives, the four horsemen of sickness: fake processed sugars, trans fats, seed oils, and food dyes. They are designed in a laboratory and are targeted to addict you, trigger cravings, and taste good. For the processors, they are cheap to mass produce and meant to increase profits from top to bottom. For deeply educated people who understand just how problematic this is, many will tell you it is catastrophic to the health, well-being, and longevity of our society. I couldn't agree more.

Sixty years ago, when most of our food supply was produced with far fewer chemicals and pesticides and our supply was closer to the natural earth, coming from organic farms and natural livestock herds, we didn't have to worry about the disgusting toxic landscape of chemical fertilizers—fake sugars, trans fats, seed oils, fake food coloring, and toxic feed used in fish farming—that we see today. These were all created in a lab to make food more visually appealing, make it grow faster, etc.

Our soils have been burned out by chemical NPK fertilizers that are a by-product of oil refining, and as a result, there is no more adequately mineralized soil to grow healthy produce in. As a result, our produce is lacking nutrient density and gets passed on to the public consumer as empty nutritional foods. These foods have very low nutritional values when compared to food from sixty years ago, along with being filled with fake sugars and trans fats. These additives have been introduced into the food chain in direct proportion to all the diseases that have flourished during that time, from obesity to ADHA and metabolic syndrome. Just look back—in the 1940s, 1950s, 1960s, and even through the 1970s, we had *none* of these diseases. They all exist because Wall Street greed and corrupt politicians allowed laws to be passed that ushered in weak and sick into society at our expense. But that's another book for another time.

Go to YouTube and search Dr. Lustig: *Sugar is poison* and Dr. Lustig: *Why everyone is sick and weak.*

These are great videos on seed oils, processed sugar, and trans fats and how they're killing you.

Dr. Lustig is one of my favorite researchers and an expert on the epidemic of toxic processed foods in our diets—i.e., obesity, insulin resistance, sugar, and trans fats. He is a neuroendocrinologist and professor at the University of California.

You'll see what I am talking about. I hope you're sitting down while you watch.

Processed Sugar Is Poison

Stop ingesting processed sugars. Now.

Sugar is a master of disguise: just because you don't see "sugar" on the ingredient list when scanning a nutrition label does not mean the item is sugar or sweetener free. There are a number of synonyms for sugar that you should be aware of—at least forty-eight of them!

Sugar goes by a slew of different names, making it easy for manufacturers to hide how much is truly in a given product. While some of these names are more obvious, like brown and cane sugar, others are trickier to spot (e.g., maltodextrin and dextrose).

Shockingly, over 68% of barcoded food products sold in the US contain added sweeteners—even if they are labeled as natural or healthy.

Sugar is sneaky and can appear where you least expect it. There are the more obvious items like cakes, sweets, sodas, and the table sugar that you might add to your morning coffee. But it can also hide out in things like sauces, salad dressings, granola bars, and pre-made foods. Even fruit—while it's considered natural—contains sugar.

Everyone's tolerance for sugar is different, but for people with type 2 diabetes who are carbohydrate intolerant, consuming too much sugar can lead to issues like spiking blood sugar, weight gain, and more. If you have a lower tolerance to carbohydrates, it's important to be aware of all of the different names, or synonyms, for sugar, so you can check labels and identify products where it might be hiding out, even when at first glance, the nutrition facts appear to show the food is low in carbs and added sugar.

The best way to ensure you're not consuming excess added sugars is to get in the habit of always scanning the ingredient list below before you throw an item in your cart. Keep in mind that ingredients are listed by quantity from high to low: the closer to the front of the list a form of sugar is, the more the product contains.

Feeling overwhelmed? You should be. Use this list of sugar names below to help you avoid a head rush when you shop!

SUGAR SYNONYMS
(The most common names for sugar,
excluding artificial sweeteners and sugar substitutes)

Basic Simple Sugars (monosaccharides and disaccharides):

Dextrose

Fructose

Galactose

Glucose

Lactose

Maltose

Sucrose

Solid or Granulated Sugars:

Beet sugar

Brown sugar

Cane juice crystals

Cane sugar

Castor sugar

Coconut sugar

Confectioner's sugar
(a.k.a. powdered sugar)

Corn syrup solids

Crystalline fructose

Date sugar

Demerara sugar

Dextrin

Diastatic malt

Ethyl maltol

Florida crystals

Golden sugar

Glucose syrup solids

Grape sugar

Icing sugar

Maltodextrin

Muscovado sugar

Panela sugar

Raw sugar

Sugar (granulated or
table)

Sucanat

Turbinado sugar

Yellow sugar

Liquid or Syrup Sugars:

Agave nectar/syrup

Barley malt

Blackstrap molasses

Brown rice syrup

Buttered
sugar/buttercream

Caramel

Carob syrup

Corn syrup

Evaporated cane juice

Fruit juice

Fruit juice concentrate

Golden syrup

High-fructose corn syrup
(HFCS)

Honey

Invert sugar   Rice syrup

Malt syrup   Refiner's syrup

Maple syrup   Sorghum syrup

Molasses   Treacle

Metabolic Rates: Energy Expenditure and Intake

There are three metabolic components involved in your caloric needs.

1. BMR – The base caloric requirement to keep you alive (no movement)

2. RMR – Additional caloric requirement that supplies all energy/movement expenditure

3. TEF – Energy required for the breakdown and transport of food

The basal metabolic rate (BMR) represents the number of calories your body needs to maintain basic physiological functions while at rest. These functions include breathing, circulation, cell production, and maintaining body temperature. BMR is influenced by factors such as age, gender, body composition, and genetics. Generally, BMR tends to decrease with age as muscle mass decreases and fat mass increases. However, regular physical activity can help maintain or even increase BMR by increasing lean muscle mass.

The resting metabolic rate (RMR) is similar to BMR but is measured under less restrictive conditions. RMR takes into account a person's physiological state while at rest but adds a higher calorie expenditure due to physical activity. It includes the energy needed for basic bodily functions as well as the energy required for digestion, absorption, and transportation of nutrients, but the real expenditure of calories via RMR comes from physical movement—e.g., resistance training, cardio training, or working a physical job. These requirements are much higher for someone like a pro fighter or a carpenter or roofer, whose job is physically demanding, compared to a clerk (who sits all day) or someone working a desk job. RMR is a very important component of total caloric expenditure. Like BMR, RMR tends to decline with age, but engaging in regular exercise can mitigate this decline, which becomes a major factor in weight management.

The thermic effect of food (TEF) represents the energy expenditure associated with the digestion, absorption, and utilization of nutrients from food. Different macronutrients have varying thermic effects—proteins have a higher TEF compared to fats and carbohydrates. TEF contributes to the total caloric expenditure, albeit to a lesser extent than BMR and RMR. The aging process typically results in a decrease in TEF due to factors such as decreased muscle mass and a potentially slower metabolism. However, a balanced diet with an appropriate distribution of macronutrients can optimize TEF.

The Age Factor

As mentioned, all three metabolic rates tend to decline with age, primarily due to changes in body composition, including reduction in muscle mass. Aging is also associated with a decrease in physical activity, which further contributes to a decline in metabolic rates. However, engaging in regular exercise, especially resistance training, can help counteract these age-related changes by preserving or increasing muscle mass and boosting metabolic rates. This is exactly why resistance and cardio training are *vital* pieces of aging strong. It is a must for longevity and quality of life!

Impact of an Active Lifestyle

A very active lifestyle, characterized by regular exercise and physical activity, has a positive impact on all three metabolic rates. Exercise, particularly strength training, can contribute to the maintenance or increase of lean muscle mass, thereby supporting higher BMR and RMR. Additionally, physical activity can enhance the TEF by promoting efficient nutrient utilization.

Metabolic Set Point

In addition to metabolic rates. It is very important to understand body composition. There are two major components of it, lean body mass and fat weight. The metabolic set point relates to an individual's BMR and how it can adapt in response to changes in diet, exercise, and body composition. It suggests that the body has a "set point" for weight and metabolism, which is regulated by various factors, including genetics, hormones, and lifestyle choices. The idea is that the body tries to maintain a stable weight by adjusting metabolism in response to changes in energy intake and expenditure. This set point can make it challenging for individuals to lose fat or gain muscle, as the body resists these changes.

Changing the metabolic set point for fat loss or muscle gain typically takes around six weeks due to the complex interplay of the factors involved. Therefore, you must be patient and think incrementally throughout your journey. Mind set and expectation management is critical.

Nutrition: Diet plays a critical role in changing the metabolic set point. When you consistently consume more calories than your body needs, it can lead to fat gain. Conversely, when you create a calorie deficit by consuming fewer calories than your body requires, it can lead to fat loss. To change the metabolic set point for fat loss, a sustained calorie deficit is essential for the right intervals and for a controlled period of time. Make sure you do *not* starve yourself to lose weight. This is one of the biggest mistakes the non-educated person makes. You will end up suffering muscle loss if you do this. To support muscle gain, a surplus of calories, primarily from protein, is necessary. The body needs time to adjust to these new calorie intakes.

Resistance Training: Muscle plays a significant role in determining the metabolic set point. The more muscle you have, the higher your BMR, as muscle tissue requires more energy to maintain than fat tissue. Resistance training stimulates muscle growth, which in turn increases BMR. To change the metabolic set point for muscle gain, a structured resistance training program is vital.

Consistency: Consistency is key when it comes to changing the metabolic set point. It takes time for the body to adapt to new dietary and exercise patterns. After a period of around six weeks, your body begins to recognize the new patterns as the new norm.

Hormonal Changes: Hormones, such as insulin and leptin, also play a role in the metabolic set point. For fat loss, reducing insulin resistance through improved diet and exercise can help the body better utilize stored fat for energy. For muscle gain, optimizing anabolic hormones like testosterone and growth hormone can support muscle development.

Adaptive Thermogenesis: The body can adapt to changes in energy intake by slowing down or speeding up metabolism. This adaptation is often seen during weight loss, where the body becomes more efficient at conserving energy. To overcome this adaptation, it's crucial to continually adjust dietary and exercise strategies.

Individual Variation: It's important to acknowledge that the rate of change in the metabolic set point can vary widely among individuals. Genetics, age, sex, and other factors all contribute to this variability.

To successfully change the metabolic set point for fat loss or muscle gain, it's essential to work with a structured and sustainable plan. It should include a well-balanced diet with the appropriate calorie intake, a regular exercise routine with a focus on resistance training, and a long-term commitment to these lifestyle changes.

Ultimately, achieving and maintaining your desired body composition is a gradual process, and it's important to be patient and consistent. The 6-week time frame is a rough estimate and can vary from person to person. However, by understanding the metabolic set point and the factors that influence it, individuals can make informed choices to reach their fitness and body composition goals effectively and sustainably.

Whole Proteins: You MUST Get These Right

This is worth covering again. Whole proteins and essential amino acids are critical components for muscle hypertrophy and protein synthesis during resistance training. Athletes, especially those engaged in strength and muscle-building activities, require an increased intake of whole dietary protein to support these processes. In my coaching experiences, where I've worked with several hundred people, I've found that protein intake is one of the pieces that people continue to get wrong even after it has been explained. You need to prioritize this part of the puzzle. Otherwise, you will be cutting yourself short on the materials that are vitally required for the muscle-building process.

Whole Proteins and Muscle Hypertrophy:

Whole proteins are dietary sources of protein that contain a broad spectrum of amino acids, including the essential amino acids (EAAs) necessary for muscle protein synthesis. Muscle hypertrophy, an increase in muscle size, is a key goal for many athletes engaged in resistance training. To achieve hypertrophy, the body requires a sufficient supply of amino acids, especially the EAAs, which the body cannot synthesize on its own.

Essential Amino Acids (EAAs):

The EAAs are a group of amino acids that must be obtained through the diet because the body cannot produce them. Among these, leucine is particularly crucial for stimulating muscle protein synthesis, as it activates the mammalian target of rapamycin (mTOR) pathway, a central regulator of muscle growth.

Increased Dietary Protein Intake for Athletes:

Research conducted by leading experts in the field of exercise physiology and nutrition consistently emphasizes the importance of increased dietary protein intake for athletes, especially during periods of resistance training. Several studies have provided valuable insights into the optimal protein intake for muscle hypertrophy.

My Personal Favorite Whole Protein Sources:

Direct farm whole eggs	Venison
Direct farm red meats	Bison
Whey protein	Turkey tenderloins
Cow liver	Pork tenderloin
Wild-caught salmon	Greek yogurt
All wild-caught fish – *never*	Cheese
farm raised (Toxic!)	Cottage cheese
Organic chicken	Raw milk
Turkey	

Red meat is a very prized high-level source of a complete protein and contains all the nine muscle-building EAAs that the body cannot produce on its own, making it a primary complete protein source for top athletes. The EAAs found in red meat that the human body *cannot* make on its own, which are not found in carbohydrates or lipid sources, are listed on page 142.

These EAAs are vital and necessary for building and repairing muscle (and all) tissues, producing enzymes and hormones, and supporting immune function, among other functions in the body.

Adequate whole protein intake/levels keep you in a positive nitrogen balance, which is a term used to describe a state in which the body retains more nitrogen than it excretes. Nitrogen is an essential component of amino acids. When the body is in a positive nitrogen balance, it indicates that there is a sufficient amount of dietary protein available for the synthesis of new proteins. In the context of building muscle mass, being in a positive nitrogen balance is crucial because it signifies that the body has an excess of amino acids available for muscle protein synthesis. This balance is necessary to support the growth, repair, and maintenance of muscle tissue and all other tissues in the body.

Muscle protein synthesis is a complex process that involves the translation of genetic information into new muscle proteins. Adequate protein intake provides the necessary amino acids to initiate and sustain this process. When protein intake is insufficient, the body may enter a negative nitrogen balance, meaning that nitrogen excretion exceeds intake. In this state, the body breaks down muscle proteins to obtain the needed amino acids, resulting in muscle protein degradation.

To achieve a positive nitrogen balance and promote muscle growth, it is important to consume an adequate amount of dietary protein. The recommended protein intake varies depending on factors such as body weight, training intensity, and individual goals. For individuals engaged in regular resistance training, the American College of Sports Medicine suggests a protein intake of approximately 1.2–2.0 grams per kilogram of body weight per day.

By consuming enough dietary protein, the body can supply the necessary amino acids for muscle protein synthesis, promoting an anabolic environment that supports muscle growth and repair. This positive nitrogen balance helps ensure that the body has a surplus of amino acids with which to build new muscle proteins, leading to muscle hypertrophy (increase in muscle size) over time.

It is worth noting that while protein intake is crucial, achieving a positive nitrogen balance alone is not sufficient for building muscle mass. Resistance training, adequate caloric intake, and a well-rounded diet that includes other essential nutrients are also important factors in supporting muscle growth.

Consulting with a registered dietitian or nutritionist can provide personalized recommendations for protein intake and overall dietary strategies to optimize muscle growth based on individual needs and goals.

Carbohydrates

Carbs get a bad rap. The good ones aren't as bad as you think. Complex carbohydrates play a crucial role in supporting protein synthesis and muscle fiber hypertrophy at the cellular level. When consumed as part of a balanced diet, complex carbohydrates provide the body with a steady supply of glucose, which serves as the primary energy source for cells, including muscle cells.

During intense exercise, such as resistance training, muscle cells require energy to perform contractions and support protein synthesis. Complex carbohydrates are broken down into glucose through digestion and absorbed into the bloodstream. This glucose is then transported to muscle cells, where it is used to produce ATP (adenosine triphosphate), the energy currency of cells.

The availability of an adequate energy supply from complex carbohydrates is vital for protein synthesis, the process by which muscle fibers are repaired and rebuilt after exercise-induced damage. Protein synthesis involves the translation of genetic information stored in DNA into proteins, the building blocks of muscle tissue.

ATP, produced from the breakdown of complex carbohydrates, provides the necessary energy for protein synthesis to occur. When energy levels are insufficient due to a lack of carbohydrates, the body may prioritize other energy-demanding processes, such as maintaining basic metabolic functions, rather than investing resources into protein synthesis. This can hinder muscle fiber hypertrophy and limit the gains achieved through resistance training.

Moreover, complex carbohydrates indirectly support protein synthesis by sparing dietary protein. When carbohydrates are inadequate, the body may rely on protein as an energy source through a process called gluconeogenesis. This means that protein, which is crucial for muscle repair and growth, may be used as an alternative energy source instead of being utilized for its intended role in protein synthesis.

By providing a consistent supply of glucose, complex carbohydrates help maintain stable blood sugar levels and prevent the breakdown of protein for energy. This allows dietary protein to be utilized primarily for its intended purpose, which is supporting muscle repair, growth, and protein synthesis.

Complex carbohydrates play a crucial role in supporting protein synthesis and maintaining energy levels in the body. They provide a sustained source of energy and the necessary building blocks for various physiological processes. Some important complex carbohydrates include:

1. **Starch:** Found in foods like grains (e.g., rice, wheat, oats), legumes (e.g., beans, lentils), and starchy vegetables (e.g., potatoes). Starches break down into glucose, providing a steady supply of energy.

2. **Fiber:** While not a direct energy source, dietary fiber from sources like whole grains, fruits, and vegetables supports overall digestive health, ensuring efficient nutrient absorption, including of protein.

3. **Glycogen:** Stored as a complex carbohydrate in the liver and muscles, glycogen acts as a reserve energy source for the body, especially during intense physical activity.

Complex carbohydrates are essential because:

- They are slowly digested, leading to a gradual release of glucose into the bloodstream, which helps maintain stable energy levels throughout the day.

- Adequate carbohydrate intake spares protein from being used as an energy source, allowing it to be primarily utilized for protein synthesis and tissue repair.

- Carbohydrates are vital for replenishing glycogen stores after exercise, ensuring optimal performance and recovery.

Lipids (fats)

In the realm of human nutrition, fats play a pivotal role, with their effects on health ranging from beneficial to detrimental. Understanding the intricacies of good fats and the harmful consequences of bad fats is crucial for crafting a balanced and wholesome diet.

Benefits of Good Fats:

Heart Health: Good fats, specifically monounsaturated and polyunsaturated fats, contribute to heart health by reducing levels of LDL cholesterol and triglycerides. They also promote a favorable lipid profile, lowering the risk of cardiovascular diseases.

Brain Function: Omega-3 fatty acids, a type of polyunsaturated fat, are essential for optimal brain function and development. They enhance cognitive performance and may reduce the risk of neurodegenerative diseases.

Cellular Structure: Saturated fats, when consumed in moderation, play a role in maintaining the structural integrity of cell membranes. They provide stability to cells and aid in various physiological functions.

Vitamin Absorption: Fats facilitate the absorption of fat-soluble vitamins (A, D, E, and K), ensuring their efficient utilization within the body. This is vital for overall health and wellness.

Energy Reserves: Fats serve as a concentrated source of energy, allowing the body to store excess calories for later use. This energy reserve is crucial during periods of fasting or increased physical activity.

Hormone Production: Certain fats are precursors to hormone synthesis. Adequate intake of these fats supports the production of hormones essential for various bodily functions, including reproduction and metabolism.

Inflammation Regulation: Omega-3 fatty acids possess anti-inflammatory properties, helping to regulate the body's inflammatory response. This is particularly beneficial in reducing the risk of chronic inflammatory conditions.

Good Fats and Sources:

Monounsaturated Fat: Olive oil, avocados, and nuts (e.g., almonds, cashews).

Polyunsaturated Fat: Fatty fish (e.g., salmon, mackerel), flaxseeds, and walnuts.

Saturated Fat (in moderation): Coconut oil, dairy products, and lean meats.

Omega-3 Fatty Acids: Fatty fish, chia seeds, and walnuts.

Harmful Effects of Bad Fats:

Increased LDL Cholesterol: Trans fats and excessive saturated fats can elevate LDL cholesterol levels, contributing to atherosclerosis and heart disease.

Inflammation: Diets rich in unhealthy fats, especially trans fats coupled with fake sugar, can promote inflammation within the body, increasing the risk of chronic diseases, such as arthritis and diabetes. This is a real health killer.

Weight Gain: Bad fats, often found in processed and fried foods, are calorie-dense and can contribute to weight gain when consumed in excess.

Impaired Blood Sugar Control: Diets high in saturated and trans fats may interfere with insulin sensitivity, potentially leading to insulin resistance and impaired blood sugar control, a precursor to type 2 diabetes.

Understanding the nuanced roles of good and bad fats empowers individuals to make informed dietary choices, promoting overall health and well-being. Balancing fat intake and choosing sources wisely contribute significantly to the prevention of various lifestyle-related diseases.

The Role and Importance of Fiber

Dietary fiber is an essential nutrient for digestive health, metabolic balance, and long-term disease prevention. Adults should aim to consume 25–38 grams of fiber daily (women: ~25g; men: ~30–38g), yet most fall short, averaging less than 15 grams per day. Fiber comes in two primary forms—soluble and insoluble—each serving distinct roles in the body.

Soluble Fiber

- **How it Works:** Dissolves in water to form a gel-like substance in the gut.

- **Sources:** Oats, beans, lentils, apples, citrus fruits, barley, psyllium.

- **Benefits:**

  o Slows digestion and absorption of carbohydrates, stabilizing blood sugar.

  o Lowers LDL cholesterol by binding to bile acids.

  o Supports satiety, reducing overeating.

  o Nourishes gut microbiota, producing beneficial short-chain fatty acids (SCFAs) like butyrate, which improve colon health and reduce inflammation.

Insoluble Fiber

- **How it Works:** Does not dissolve in water; adds bulk to stool and speeds passage through the intestines.

- **Sources:** Whole grains, nuts, seeds, vegetables (carrots, cauliflower, green beans), wheat bran.

- **Benefits:**

  o Promotes regular bowel movements and prevents constipation.

- o Helps maintain healthy colon function and lowers risk of diverticulitis.
- o Contributes to satiety by increasing meal volume.

Why Both Matter

- **Balanced Health:** Together, soluble and insoluble fibers reduce the risk of cardiovascular disease, type 2 diabetes, obesity, and certain cancers.

- **Longevity Impact:** Adequate fiber intake improves gut health, metabolic control, and resilience against age-related decline—making it a cornerstone of lifelong vitality.

Top 10 Fiber-Rich Foods

1. Lentils (15g per cup, cooked)
2. Black beans (15g per cup, cooked)
3. Split peas (16g per cup, cooked)
4. Chickpeas (12g per cup, cooked)
5. Avocado (10g per medium fruit)
6. Raspberries (8g per cup)
7. Pear (6g per medium fruit)
8. Oats (8g per cup, cooked)
9. Chia seeds (10g per ounce / 2 Tbsp)
10. Almonds (4g per ounce / ~23 nuts)

MICRONUTRIENTS – MINERALS AND VITAMINS

As we have discussed, proteins, carbohydrates, and fats are the core macronutrients that fuel the body, while micronutrients—vitamins and minerals—support countless vital functions. An adequate, well-balanced diet that includes both is essential for maintaining strong health and overall well-being.

When you embark on a proper fitness program like The FITNESS QUADRANT, your requirement for all nutrients becomes much higher. You need to scale up your nutrition amount to meet the metabolic demand that gets triggered during workouts. Sufficient levels of both major and minor minerals are vital for maintaining various physiological processes in the body, including supporting an anabolic state necessary for muscle growth and overall health. These minerals are essential for enzymatic reactions, nerve function, muscle contraction, fluid balance, and maintaining the structural integrity of various tissues.

Major minerals, also known as macro-minerals, are required in larger amounts by the body.

Minor minerals, also known as trace minerals, are required in smaller amounts by the body.

These minerals play critical roles in maintaining various biochemical reactions and physiological processes that support overall health and anabolic state. They are involved in energy production, protein synthesis, cellular signaling, immune function, and structural support.

To maintain an optimum level of functioning, it is important to consume a well-balanced diet that provides adequate amounts of both major and minor minerals.

Essential Minerals and Their Functions:

1. **Calcium:** Vital for bone and teeth formation, blood clotting, and muscle function. Sources include dairy products, leafy greens, and fortified foods.

2. **Phosphorus:** Works in tandem with calcium for bone health, contributes to energy metabolism, and forms a part of DNA and RNA. Found in dairy, meat, and whole grains.

3. **Potassium:** Crucial for maintaining fluid balance, nerve impulses, and muscle contractions. Abundant in bananas, oranges, potatoes, and leafy greens.

4. **Sodium:** Regulates fluid balance, nerve function, and muscle contractions. Commonly found in table salt and processed foods.

5. **Magnesium:** Essential for muscle and nerve function, bone health, and energy production. Nuts, seeds, leafy greens, and whole grains are excellent sources.

6. **Iron:** Required for oxygen transport in the blood, energy metabolism, and immune function. Found in red meat, poultry, beans, and fortified cereals.

7. **Zinc:** Supports immune function, wound healing, and DNA synthesis. Sources include meat, dairy, nuts, and legumes.

8. **Copper:** Plays a role in iron metabolism, connective tissue formation, and antioxidant defense. Nuts, seeds, whole grains, and seafood are good sources.

9. **Selenium:** Acts as an antioxidant, supporting immune function and thyroid health. Found in Brazil nuts, seafood, and whole grains.

10. **Iodine:** Essential for thyroid hormone production, crucial for metabolism and growth. Seafood and iodized salt are common sources.

11. **Manganese:** Contributes to bone formation, blood clotting, and antioxidant defense. Nuts, seeds, whole grains, and leafy greens are rich in manganese.

12. **Chromium:** Aids in insulin function, contributing to glucose metabolism. Broccoli, whole grains, and lean meats are good sources.

13. **Molybdenum:** Supports enzyme function and metabolism. Found in legumes, nuts, and whole grains.

Vitamins and Their Functions:

1. **Vitamin A:** Essential for vision, immune function, and skin health. Sources include sweet potatoes, carrots, and dark leafy greens.

2. **Vitamin B1 (Thiamine):** Supports energy metabolism and nerve function. Found in whole grains, pork, and beans.

3. **Vitamin B2 (Riboflavin):** Facilitates energy production and antioxidant defense. Dairy products, lean meats, and leafy greens are sources.

4. **Vitamin B3 (Niacin):** Vital for energy metabolism and DNA repair. Meat, fish, and whole grains contain niacin.

5. **Vitamin B5 (Pantothenic Acid):** Contributes to energy metabolism and hormone synthesis. Present in meat, dairy, and whole grains.

6. **Vitamin B6 (Pyridoxine):** Involved in amino acid metabolism and neurotransmitter synthesis. Sources include poultry, fish, and bananas.

7. **Vitamin B7 (Biotin):** Supports metabolism and skin health. Eggs, nuts, and sweet potatoes are good biotin sources.

8. **Vitamin B9 (Folate):** Essential for DNA synthesis and cell division. Found in leafy greens, legumes, and fortified grains.

9. **Vitamin B12 (Cobalamin):** Crucial for nerve function and red blood cell production. Present in animal products and fortified foods.

10. **Vitamin C (Ascorbic Acid):** Acts as an antioxidant, supports immune function, and aids in collagen synthesis. Citrus fruits, berries, and bell peppers are rich in vitamin C.

11. **Vitamin D:** Necessary for calcium absorption, bone health, and immune function. Sun exposure, fatty fish, and fortified dairy products are sources.

12. **Vitamin E (Tocopherol):** An antioxidant that protects cells from damage. Nuts, seeds, and vegetable oils contain vitamin E.

13. **Vitamin K:** Essential for blood clotting and bone health. Leafy greens, broccoli, and soybean oil are good sources.

Whole Food Sources of Vitamins:

1. **Leafy Greens:** Spinach, kale, and Swiss chard are rich in various vitamins and minerals, including calcium, iron, and vitamins A and K.

2. **Nuts and Seeds:** Almonds, walnuts, sunflower seeds, and flaxseeds provide a mix of vitamins (E, B) and minerals (magnesium, zinc).

3. **Fruits:** Citrus fruits (oranges, lemons) offer vitamin C, while bananas and avocados provide potassium and B vitamins.

4. **Dairy Products:** Milk, yogurt, and cheese are excellent sources of calcium, vitamin D, and B vitamins.

5. **Fish:** Fatty fish, like salmon and mackerel, are rich in omega-3 fatty acids, vitamin D, and minerals like phosphorus.

6. **Meat:** Lean meats such as poultry and lean beef are sources of protein, iron, zinc, and B vitamins.

7. **Whole Grains:** Brown rice, quinoa, and oats provide a variety of vitamins (B, E) and minerals (magnesium, phosphorus).

8. **Legumes:** Beans, lentils, and chickpeas offer a mix of vitamins (B, folate) and minerals (iron, zinc).

9. **Vegetables:** Broccoli, carrots, sweet potatoes, and bell peppers contribute to a diverse nutrient profile, including vitamins A and C.

10. **Eggs:** A source of protein, vitamin B12, and biotin.

Including a wide variety of these whole foods in a balanced diet ensures an adequate intake of essential minerals and vitamins, promoting overall health and preventing nutritional deficiencies.

C = CARDIOVASCULAR
(bottom left quadrant)

This is where your heart and lungs are strengthened, and fat is burned. During cardiovascular exercise, such as running, cycling, or swimming, the body's demand for oxygen and energy increases. To meet this increased demand, the heart pumps blood more vigorously, resulting in an elevated heart rate. In order to obtain optimal benefits for brain-derived neurotrophic factor (BDNF) release and to subsequently enhance brain health, it's recommended that people exercise within a specific heart rate zone, typically between 70% and 80% of your maximum heart rate.

The maximum heart rate is an individual's maximum achievable heart rate during physical exertion and can be estimated using the formula: maximum heart rate (MHR) = 220 – age. For example, for a 30-year-old individual, their estimated maximum heart rate would be 190 beats per minute (bpm) using this formula.

Exercising within the 70% to 80% of MHR range ensures that the cardiovascular system is adequately stimulated and the body experiences moderate-intensity exercise. This level of intensity is beneficial for the release of BDNF. When an individual engages in cardiovascular exercise within this heart rate zone, it triggers a cascade of physiological responses, including the release of BDNF. For the same 30-year-old person, the bpm would then be 190 x 72% (and up to 80%) which equals 137 bpm when doing their cardio bouts.

BDNF is a protein that plays a crucial role in supporting the growth, survival, and maintenance of neurons (nerve cells) in the brain. BDNF is released in response to various stimuli, including cardiovascular exercise. BDNF has become a promising (and heavily studied) component of fighting the battle of early dementia and Alzheimer's disease. This is *exactly* why proper fitness systems need to be deployed throughout your life.

BDNF is released in response to stressors experienced during exercise. It acts as a neuroprotective and neurotrophic factor, enhancing the growth, function, and survival of neurons in the brain. BDNF supports the formation of new neural connections (synaptogenesis), enhances synaptic plasticity (the ability of the brain to reorganize and adapt), and promotes the survival of existing neurons (neuroprotection). These processes are critical for learning, memory, and overall cognitive function.

Regular cardiovascular exercise that triggers the release of BDNF helps to maintain a healthy brain throughout a person's lifespan. It's associated with improved cognitive function, enhanced mood, reduced risk of neurodegenerative diseases such as Alzheimer's and Parkinson's, and an overall healthier brain structure.

Engaging in cardiovascular exercise within the 70% to 80% of maximum heart rate range promotes the release of BDNF. This is also the ideal bpm range for accessing fat (yellow adipose tissue) for fuel during your cardio bout, along with optimal fat-burning zone.

Heart, Lungs, and Blood Pressure

Cardiovascular exercise, performed within the target heart rate zone of 70% to 80% of an individual's maximum heart rate, has profound effects on both the lungs and the heart, leading to strengthening of the respiratory and cardiovascular systems.

1. **Lung Strengthening:**

   Cardiovascular exercise significantly strengthens the respiratory system, particularly the lungs. During exercise within the recommended heart rate zone, the body demands more oxygen to fuel muscles and other tissues. This increased demand for oxygen triggers the lungs to work harder and more efficiently. The respiratory muscles, including the diaphragm and intercostal muscles, become stronger and more resilient due to the consistent demand for deep breathing and increased oxygen intake. Over time, this leads to improved lung capacity, increased efficiency of oxygen exchange, and enhanced respiratory endurance, allowing individuals to sustain physical activity for longer durations.

2. **Heart Muscle Myocardial Wall Thickness Increase:**

   Regular cardiovascular exercise also induces positive adaptations in the heart muscle, known as the myocardium. The myocardial walls of the heart thicken in response to the increased workload imposed by cardiovascular exercise. When exercising within the 70% to 80% of MHR, the heart pumps blood more vigorously to supply muscles and organs with oxygen and nutrients. This increased pumping action leads to hypertrophy (enlargement) of the heart's ventricular walls, particularly the left ventricle, which is responsible for pumping oxygenated blood throughout the body. The thicker myocardial walls enhance the heart's efficiency and ability to pump blood effectively, improving overall cardiovascular function and endurance.

3. **Blood Pressure Reduction:**

   Engaging in cardiovascular exercise within the specified heart rate zone contributes to better management of blood pressure. Regular exercise strengthens the heart, enabling it to pump blood more efficiently with each contraction. This efficiency reduces the resistance the blood encounters as it flows through arteries, ultimately leading to a drop in blood pressure.

Consistent cardiovascular exercise promotes vasodilation (widening of blood vessels), allowing for smoother blood flow and lower systemic blood pressure levels, both during exercise and at rest. Additionally, exercise stimulates the release of nitric oxide, a vasodilator, which further aids in maintaining healthy blood pressure levels.

4. **Resting Heart Rate Reduction:**

   Regular cardiovascular exercise within the prescribed heart rate zone helps in lowering the resting heart rate, the number of heart beats per minute when the body is at rest. The heart becomes more efficient at pumping blood with each beat, requiring fewer beats to meet the body's needs. The increased efficiency is a result of the heart's adaptation to consistent exercise, leading to a stronger stroke volume (amount of blood pumped per beat). As a consequence, the heart doesn't need to beat as frequently at rest to maintain adequate blood circulation, resulting in a lower resting heart rate.

To summarize, exercising within the 70% to 80% of maximum heart rate range is the optimal fat-burning range while you train, and this range also brings about positive adaptations in both the respiratory and cardiovascular systems. The lungs strengthen through improved capacity and efficiency (they adapt to the stress), while the heart muscle's myocardial walls thicken to enhance pumping efficiency (a stronger heart lowers resting heart rate). Furthermore, cardiovascular exercise in this heart rate range helps in reducing blood pressure and resting heart rate, contributing to an overall healthier cardiovascular profile and improved physical well-being.

Increased Capillary Density

This benefit is *never* talked about in mainstream America. Why? Because the knowledge level overall—including that of certified trainers—is virtually nonexistent. Cardiovascular exercise, especially when sustained for at least thirty minutes at the specified heart rate zone, triggers an increase in capillary density within muscles.

Capillaries are the smallest blood vessels in the body, and they play a critical role in facilitating the exchange of nutrients, oxygen, and waste products between the blood and muscle cells. Regular exercise, particularly aerobic activities, prompts the body to adapt to the increased demand for oxygen and nutrients during prolonged physical exertion. In response, the body generates more capillaries around muscle fibers, creating a denser network. This enhanced capillary density ensures efficient nutrient and oxygen delivery to muscle tissues during exercise.

Enhanced Mitochondrial Density

Again, this benefit is *never* talked about in mainstream America. Why? Because the knowledge level overall is, again, virtually nonexistent.

Cardiovascular exercise performed within the target heart rate zone has a significant impact on the body's capillary and mitochondrial density, leading to numerous physiological benefits.

Mitochondria are the powerhouse of cells, responsible for generating adenosine triphosphate (ATP), the primary energy currency of the cell. Cardiovascular exercise at the recommended heart rate zone stimulates the growth and proliferation of mitochondria within muscle cells. Mitochondria are essential for aerobic metabolism, where oxygen is used to produce ATP through cellular respiration. The increased demand for energy during sustained cardiovascular exercise prompts the body to create more mitochondria to meet this energy need. The higher mitochondrial density translates to improved ATP production, enabling enhanced endurance and prolonged physical performance.

Significance of Mitochondria and Capillaries for ATP and Stem Cell Storage

Mitochondria are central to the production of ATP, the molecule that stores and releases energy for cellular processes. The increase in mitochondrial density due to consistent cardiovascular exercise means the body can store more ATP, providing a greater reservoir of readily available energy for muscle contractions and sustained activity. Stem cells, vital for tissue repair and regeneration, also benefit from enhanced capillary and mitochondrial density. Capillaries provide an avenue for the distribution of stem cells to different tissues in the body, facilitating tissue repair and growth. Having more capillaries means there is an efficient transport system to carry stem cells to areas where they are needed for regeneration and repair.

Improved Oxygen Delivery and Waste Product Removal

The increased capillary density resulting from regular cardiovascular exercise ensures efficient delivery of oxygen to muscle cells during physical activity. Oxygen is essential for the cellular processes that produce energy, and a well-developed capillary network supports the delivery of this vital element. Additionally, more capillaries aid in the removal of waste products, such as carbon dioxide and lactic acid, from muscle cells. This efficient waste removal helps delay fatigue during exercise, allowing for longer and more sustained physical effort.

In summary, consistent cardiovascular exercise within the 70% to 80% of maximum heart rate range leads to a significant increase in both capillary and mitochondrial density. These adaptations have far-reaching benefits, including improved ATP and stem cell storage, enhanced oxygen delivery, and efficient waste product removal. Ultimately, these physiological changes contribute to enhanced endurance, better tissue repair, and improved overall performance during physical activities.

R = RECOVERY
(bottom right quadrant)

This is where you recharge your entire system, relax, and have fun with your friends or diving in to a cool hobby. Recovery is an essential component of fitness training, allowing the body to repair, adapt, and grow stronger after the stress of exercise. Without proper recovery periods, athletes risk overtraining, declining performance, and increased injury probability.

Three vitally important pieces of recovery:

1. Post-resistance workout recovery nutrition

2. Adequate daily nutrition

3. Sufficient sleep

The post-resistance training workout recovery period (45-minute window following workout) is a little-known dynamic opportunity that delivers massive results for you. It is a huge piece of the puzzle of our FITNESS QUADRANT system to trigger and stimulate muscle growth. After an adequate training session, we are depleted of ATP-CP. Remember, these are the energy compounds stored in mitochondria, which are responsible for immediate explosive muscle contractions. Post workout, muscle glycogen levels are also reduced, and the rise of cortisol levels (and other catabolic hormones) cause a heightened catabolic state. Catabolic means decay. This is the opposite of what we want, which is anabolic, a state of growth. Furthermore, the muscle damage that has occurred during exercise has stimulated an inflammatory response, which is normal because of the resistance and damage imposed on the muscle.

To keep this simple, following a resistance training bout, we are in a catabolic state for hours. This is not good. However, through science—albeit a science most are unfamiliar with—we now know that we can turn this into a major anabolic phase. The muscle is primed to shift into such a state provided you feed yourself the right nutrients within the 45-minute window following your workout. At no other time during the course of your day can nutrition make such an impact on your training program and desired results.

Immediately following your workout, consuming a post-workout drink that is a combination of sugars (fruit juice—grape juice is my preference) and whey protein (powder) in the ratio of 4 parts carb and 1 part protein will turn the anabolic switch on. This will provide your body with a serious trigger from catabolic, shifting into a major anabolic protein synthesis state that is three times higher than a normal muscle-building state. Again, I cannot stress enough that the drink needs to be ingested immediately after you work out. I mean within minutes of finishing a resistance training bout. This will multiply the muscle-building process, as you stimulate the anabolic machinery in your body by giving it the right nutrients (carb-protein drink) at the right time (post workout) as the body kicks into gear remodeling the muscle. This is one of the very few times a high-glycemic, sugar-based drink is necessary to stimulate insulin response. This is growth!

The drink I make before I head to the gym is made up of one cup of grape juice (38g carbs) diluted with a little water and one tablespoon of whey protein powder (10g) mixed in my shaker bottle with ice. There is also a post-workout recovery drink I use called Endurox R4. It is THE gold standard and embodies the science I've described, which is backed by loads of research and white papers. It's mentioned in the supplement section of this book.

Proper nutrition and sleep are both major components of recovery. Some say sleep is the most important part of successful recovery. We've all been there—having suffered a bad night's sleep or sleep deprivation. It sucks. We need a minimum of six hours every night, and even that is not really enough. Seven hours is good, eight hours is optimal.

I highly recommend the book *Why We Sleep* by Mathew Walker, PhD. It is one of the best reads you'll ever find on the importance and science of sleep.

Importance of Recovery for Muscle and Nervous System Health

1. Tissue Repair and Growth:

    o Exercise, especially resistance training, causes microtears in muscle fibers.

    o Recovery allows the body to repair these tears, leading to stronger, more resilient muscles (hypertrophy).

    o Key recovery processes, like protein synthesis, peak during rest periods.

2. Central Nervous System (CNS) Recovery:

   o High-intensity training taxes the CNS, which coordinates muscle contractions and motor skills.

   o Prolonged stress without rest can lead to CNS fatigue, reducing performance, reaction time, and strength output.

The Consequences of Overtraining

1. Declining Gains:

   o Overtraining occurs when the balance between training and recovery is disrupted.

   o Signs include decreased strength, slower recovery, poor sleep, and increased fatigue.

   o Instead of improving, performance declines due to insufficient recovery.

2. Injury Risk:

   o Overtraining increases the likelihood of muscle strains, joint injuries, and tendon overuse syndromes.

   o Persistent fatigue also compromises form and technique, further elevating injury risk.

Structured Recovery: Microcycles and Macrocycles

1. Microcycle:

   o A short training phase, typically lasting one to two weeks.

   o Focuses on specific goals, such as strength, endurance, or recovery.

   o Recovery days or light training sessions are strategically built into microcycles to balance load and rest.

2. Macrocycle:

○ A longer training phase, often spanning a few months or even a year, when aligned with major performance goals (e.g., competitions).

○ Includes multiple microcycles and planned deload weeks— periods of reduced intensity to allow full recovery.

Optimizing Recovery for Peak Performance

1. **Sleep:** Essential for muscle repair, hormonal regulation (e.g., growth hormone), and CNS recovery.

2. **Nutrition:** Adequate protein, carbohydrates, and hydration support tissue repair and energy replenishment. Post-workout nutrient-timing drink 4:1 ratio of carbs to protein.

3. **Active Recovery:** Light activities like stretching, yoga, or low-intensity cardio improve circulation and speed up recovery.

4. **Deloading:** Regularly scheduled lighter training weeks prevent burnout and maintain long-term performance gains.

By incorporating well-planned recovery phases within micro- and macrocycles, athletes and non-athletes alike can enhance performance, reduce injury risk, and sustain long-term progress. Recovery is not a break from training—it is a critical part of the process.

Recovery periods play a crucial role in optimizing performance and promoting overall well-being, especially during extreme fitness practices such as resistance and cardiovascular training. These recovery periods are essential for allowing the body to repair and adapt to the stress imposed by intense workouts, ultimately leading to enhanced physical fitness and reduced risk of injury.

One of the key components of effective recovery is sufficient sleep. During sleep, the body undergoes various physiological processes that are essential for recovery. The sleep cycle consists of different stages, including REM (rapid eye movement) and non-REM stages. During deep sleep, the body releases growth hormone, which is instrumental in muscle repair and growth. Additionally, the immune system is more active during sleep, contributing to overall recovery and strengthening the body's defense mechanisms.

In the context of resistance training, adequate sleep becomes paramount as it facilitates the repair of microtears in muscle fibers caused by intense workouts. With cardiovascular training, sleep allows the heart rate to normalize and the cardiovascular system to recover from the strain of intense aerobic exercise.

Massage work is another effective method for aiding recovery. Massages can help reduce muscle soreness, improve blood circulation, and enhance flexibility. The manipulation of soft tissues during a massage can also alleviate tension and promote a sense of relaxation, contributing to overall recovery.

Sauna time is yet another recovery strategy that has gained popularity. Saunas induce sweating, which helps eliminate toxins from the body and promotes circulation. The heat exposure during sauna sessions can also improve cardiovascular function and reduce muscle stiffness. However, it's essential to stay hydrated during sauna sessions to prevent dehydration.

Red light therapy saunas combine the benefits of infrared heat with red and near-infrared light to promote recovery, longevity, and overall wellness. This therapy penetrates deep into the skin and muscles, stimulating cellular repair and increasing blood circulation.

Key benefits of red light therapy saunas:

- **Enhanced Muscle Recovery** – Reduces inflammation and speeds up post-workout recovery.

- **Increased Collagen Production** – Improves skin elasticity and reduces wrinkles.

- **Boosted Mitochondrial Function** – Supports energy production at the cellular level.

- **Reduced Joint Pain and Inflammation** – Helps with arthritis, stiffness, and mobility.

- **Detoxification** – Sweating helps remove toxins while improving circulation.

- **Improved Sleep and Hormonal Balance** – Supports melatonin production and reduces stress.

A red light therapy sauna is an excellent tool for athletes, fitness enthusiasts, and anyone looking to enhance recovery, longevity, and performance.

Recovery periods are integral to adequate fitness practices, ensuring that the body has the opportunity to heal, adapt, and grow stronger. Incorporating sufficient sleep, proper nutrition, massage work, and sauna time into a comprehensive recovery plan can significantly enhance the effectiveness of resistance and cardiovascular training, leading to improved performance and long-term health benefits.

Fasting: Benefits and Dangers

PROPER fasting can be part of a planned recovery plan if implemented correctly once a quarter. While there are scientific benefits to fasting and it's all the rage in places, it also comes with major risks. I am personally not a big fan of fasting. I don't like being hangry. And the thought of potential muscle loss goes against what I also know to be a major scientific benefit for longevity. I work hard for my muscles, and I don't want to lose them! However, fasting can be beneficial if incorporated properly and not overused. Again, I'm just not a big fan, and I have seen people obsessed with losing weight abuse fasting and end up losing significant muscle mass instead.

A typical fast means water only for the entire period. There are also other types of fasting that involves supplemental additives for waste removal, etc., and maybe drinking beef broth or chicken broth every twelve hours during the fast.

1. **Benefits of 24-Hour and 72-Hour Fasting Protocols**

   Fasting protocols such as 24-hour, 48-hour, and 72-hour fasts have gained attention for their potential health benefits, particularly through the activation of autophagy, a cellular repair process critical for health and longevity.

- **Autophagy Activation:** During fasting, the body initiates autophagy, where cells remove their damaged components, recycle proteins, and eliminate toxins. This process is associated with:

  o **Reduced Inflammation:** Autophagy reduces pro-inflammatory cytokines, potentially lowering the risk of chronic conditions like heart disease and diabetes.

  o **Improved Cellular Health:** Autophagy facilitates the removal of dysfunctional mitochondria, which enhances energy efficiency.

  o **Neuroprotection:** Studies suggest autophagy supports brain health by clearing protein aggregates linked to neurodegenerative diseases, like Alzheimer's and Parkinson's.

- **Metabolic Benefits:**

  o **Insulin Sensitivity:** Fasting can improve insulin sensitivity and lower blood sugar levels.

  o **Fat Loss:** Depletion of glycogen stores promotes fat utilization for energy, aiding weight loss.

  o **Growth Hormone Boost:** Fasting elevates growth hormone levels, which help maintain muscle mass during calorie restriction.

- **Immune System Reset:** Extended fasting (72 hours) has been shown to regenerate immune cells by clearing out damaged ones and triggering stem cell activity, as evidenced by a study in *Cell Stem Cell* (2014).

2. Risks of Over-Fasting: Muscle Loss and Other Concerns

While fasting has numerous benefits, excessive fasting or prolonged calorie deficits can have detrimental effects, particularly on muscle mass.

- **Muscle Loss Risks:**
  - After glycogen depletion, the body may begin breaking down muscle protein for gluconeogenesis (conversion of amino acids into glucose), especially during fasts that extend beyond 48–72 hours.
  - Chronic fasting without adequate refeeding can reduce lean body mass, impair physical strength, and slow metabolism.
  - Research shows that muscle protein breakdown increases significantly if fasting is paired with low protein intake or extreme caloric restriction over time.

- **Hormonal Dysregulation:**
  - Over-fasting may suppress thyroid hormone levels (T3), leading to a slower metabolism.
  - Fasting can cause cortisol levels to rise, further promoting muscle breakdown and increasing stress.

- **Nutrient Deficiency:** Extended fasting without proper preparation and refeeding risks depleting electrolytes (e.g., sodium, potassium, magnesium), causing fatigue, heart arrhythmias, and/or cramping.

3. Finding the Balance: Practical Recommendations

- **24-Hour Fasting Protocols:** Ideal for promoting autophagy, improving insulin sensitivity, and supporting metabolic health without significant muscle loss. A quarterly protocol is sustainable for most people as long as increased protein is incorporated before and after fast.

However, *never* start fasting right after resistance training. The fast needs to be timed three days after your last resistance session.

- **48–72-Hour Fasting Protocols:** Beneficial for immune system regeneration and deep cellular repair but should be limited to occasional use (e.g., once every six months) to avoid muscle loss.

- **Strength Training and Refeeding:** Incorporating resistance training and prioritizing high-quality protein intake (2.0g/kg body weight) during refeeding (after the fast) helps preserve muscle mass and supports recovery.

- **Avoid Chronic Fasting:** Long-term repetitive fasting (e.g., weekly or multi-day fasts without adequate nutrition) is dangerous. It increases the risk of muscle wasting and metabolic adaptation. This is the obsession part that is oh so dangerous.

Fasting, when used appropriately, offers unique health benefits, especially by activating autophagy. However, excessive fasting or improper refeeding can lead to excessive muscle loss and other health issues. A balanced approach, combining fasting (maximum once per quarter) with proper nutrition and resistance training, ensures maximum benefits while minimizing risks.

CHAPTER 3

BASIC PROGRAMMING DESIGN

Make sure to always have a checkup
with your doctor before you
start any fitness program.

It is very important to point out that there are many different individual levels of fitness, from beginners (who've never trained before) to pro athletes (who have constantly trained throughout their careers). If we put a scale to this spread—say 1 to 10—then the entry point into a fitness program would mirror that same scale. This means that for the beginners (1), the onboarding plan would be heavy on explaining basic kinesiology, and very heavy on exercise form (biomechanics), followed by exercise selection, patterns, intensity, volume, etc. For a pro athlete, we would come in hot after analyzing sport-specific movements and weak points in their game, going all the way down the line into nutrition and cardiovascular programming. The point is, fitness belongs to everyone, and there is an appropriate entry point for everyone. This can sometimes be an intimidating factor and keeps a vast majority of beginners away from starting a life-changing journey into proper fitness routines. Don't let that happen to you.

YOUR FITNESS QUADRANT EXAMPLE

Now you've read about The FITNESS QUADRANT, with its four phases of fitness that all work in combination to produce unbelievable results that last. Each part of the quadrant can be dialed up or down, depending on your desired outcome. Each part has its own drop-down list, with Resistance being the most complex quadrant, followed by Nutrition. Cardiovascular is straightforward, unless you are a high-level athlete looking to shave off seconds in your event. Then cardio protocols become very scientific in terms of training systems and testing. Lastly, Recovery is also straightforward for most people. Again, if you're a high-level competitive athlete, then recovery takes on a whole other meaning and level with deeper exercise and nutritional science protocols and structure.

For the purposes of this book, we will stick to a basic resistance and cardio training design and a basic nutrition example. Understand that the resistance training protocols we use are complex and custom fit for all of our private clients based on their intended outcomes. We have hundreds of different movements and patterns that get complex with our private clients, which range from kettlebell and heavy ball functional training to compound plyometric work to modified sled and sprint intervals. We have had incredible success, with a 98%-win rate on clients hitting and exceeding their goals with The FITNESS QUADRANT system. Even doing the following basic exercises properly will deliver huge results.

Let's take an average 55-year-old person who weighs between 190–215 pounds looking to lose about 15–25 pounds of fat weight (not muscle weight!) and gain strength so they can play more golf, tennis, or pickleball at a higher level. They're also feeling more and more stiff in their lower back, knees, and particularly shoulders because every time they've gone to the gym in the past, they end up "tweaking" them. They work full time and have two kids—12 and 16.

Here is what a basic weekly program schedule would look like for them:

Resistance: 2–3 times per week, total body

Cardio: 2–3 times per week, steady state to hit fat-burning bpm

Nutrition: 3 meals per day, plus healthy snacks as needed

Recovery: 2–3 days per week

I would call this a 2-2-3 schedule (2R, 2C, 3N). The next phase might look like this: 3-3-3. Or if we were after a lot of muscle and strength gain, it would look like this: 5-1-5.

Resistance

Two to three workouts per week – 45-minute total body sessions.

We would focus on the three major muscle groups (legs, back, chest), then secondary muscles (triceps, biceps, shoulders), and then stabilizers (core, hips). I have literally hundreds of different movements (and modifications to these movements) I utilize depending on the client, and again, the desired outcome. Our range of clients is very wide. We work with people from youth sports teams and college teams and individual clients up to 85 years old—who quite frankly are loving it and kicking ass!

Here are just eight basic movements. We have hundreds of exercises in our arsenal that we utilize in very specific patterns for our clients that trigger life-changing results. If you just did these basic exercises two to three times per week *with the correct form and correct weight* that targets a 10–15 rep range—meaning on the 10th or 15th rep you are barely able to finish with correct form—you would be very far down the road of building muscle (hypertrophy) and triggering your growth mode.

You would do movements 1–4 and repeat three times through, then move on to movements 5–8 and repeat three times through. This would be 24 total sets, which you would accomplish in about 45 minutes or less. A sedentary beginner might go through them two times to start to get familiarized with the movements. Then you'd dial it up every week to three times through (or even four times through) with increased resistance loads as you progress. You could do this in your living room or basement. All you need is a TRX-type band ($60 Amazon) and some kettlebells ($100 Amazon). Get moving.

ROTATION #1 – Go through exercises 1–4 three to four times in sequence, should take about 4 to 5 minutes to complete one round and about 20 to 25 minutes to complete four total rounds.

1. Squat – various choices (DB, TRX, kettlebell, barbell)

2. Push-up or bench press

3. Row – TRX, dumbbell, or cable row

4. Core work – sit-up

Then move on to rotation #2

ROTATION #2 – Go through exercises 5–8 three to four times

1. Dead lift – sumo, barbell

2. DB shoulder press

3. DB curl

4. Triceps – TRX band, cables, decline dumbbells

Scan this QR code for a video on these eight movements:

Mobility – Your Ticket to Long-Lasting Joint Health and Free Movement

Incorporating mobility exercises into a comprehensive fitness regimen is essential for maintaining and enhancing *joint health, flexibility, and overall functional movement*. Mobility movements focus on actively engaging joints through their full range of motion, which not only improves performance but also reduces the risk of injury. Resistance training targets muscle with much higher loads, which are needed to trigger and stimulate muscle growth, as we have previously discussed.

Impact of Aging and Lack of Mobility Training

As we age, our joints often become stiffer and less flexible due to decreased synovial fluid and thinning cartilage. Ligaments may also shorten and lose elasticity, contributing to a reduced range of motion. Aging can lead to a significant decrease in muscle strength—up to 50% between the ages of 25 and 80—impairing effective body movement and daily functioning. However, studies have shown that older adults can improve flexibility and joint function through regular stretching and mobility exercises. Engaging in such activities can enhance muscle performance, balance, and confidence in movement.

Benefits of Regular Mobility Exercises

Incorporating mobility exercises into your daily routines offers several advantages:

- **Enhanced Neural Activation:** Mobility exercises stimulate neural activity within muscles, making them more effective at generating force during physical activities.

- **Improved Joint Function:** Regular mobility work increases the production of synovial fluid, reducing friction within joints and promoting smoother movements.

- **Stress Reduction:** Engaging in mobility routines can alleviate stress and promote a sense of well-being.

The FITNESS QUADRANT system integrates mobility training within its resistance training quadrant, recognizing that strength without mobility can lead to imbalances and potential injuries. By combining resistance exercises with dedicated mobility movements, this approach ensures that individuals develop strength alongside flexibility and joint integrity, leading to more balanced and effective fitness outcomes.

Incorporating mobility exercises into your fitness routine is crucial for maintaining joint health, preventing age-related decline in movement, and enhancing overall physical performance. Even a basic mobility routine can lead to significant improvements in joint integrity and functional ability. There are literally hundreds of mobility movements. Here are a few for you to watch.

Scan this QR code for a video on basic mobility movements:

Cardio

Always check with your healthcare provider to get clearance on any exercise program.

I highly recommend buying a heart rate monitor. This is a fantastic investment that helps you stay in the right heart rate zone for burning fat. Amazon has lots of choices—I recommend a model with a heart strap that connects to your phone via Bluetooth.

Basic weekly routine:

There are all different types of cardio training that require different strategies depending on the intended outcome. A marathon runner has completely different training protocols compared to a sprinter or a triathlete. Even within the sprinter's ecosystem, you have different training protocols for the 100-meter, 200-meter, or certainly the 400-meter up to 1,000-meter. You get the point; it's loaded with scientific data and methods that have been studied intensively.

For our purposes, we will cover the most common cardio training method that is utilized for fat burning, which is typically done at a constant heart rate (bpm) for an extended period of time—usually around thirty minutes. Here is a basic starting point for your cardio workouts, which are separate from your resistance workouts. If you want to combine them in the same day as your resistance workouts to become ultra-efficient in your time usage, do your resistance workout first, then your cardio bout.

I recommend the stair stepper or Jacob's ladder or a treadmill, cardio machines that can be found at most gyms. They are easy on the joints compared to running, which can aggravate or trigger foot/ankle/knee pain and/or lower back pain. If you have a treadmill, ramp it up to the highest incline so you are walking uphill. If you choose running as your preferred cardio, make sure you have high-quality running shoes, and if you can, run on a soft surface, like hard beach sand or a track that has a rubber surface. This will help lower the impact on your joints.

No matter what machine you're using, or if you are speed walking or running, it's heart rate that is important. It is measured by bpm, or beats per minute. This is where your strap will show the data and take the guess work or manual calculations out of the equation for you.

Optimal fat-burning heart rate equation:

220 – age x 72%–80% = targeted bpm for burning-fat zone

Example: for a 60-year-old, it would look like this:

220 – 60 = 160 MHR x 72%–80% = 115 bpm–128 bpm

This means you want to get your heart rate up to 128 bpm and hold it there for at least twenty minutes, preferably for over thirty minutes. As your heart gets stronger (after all, your heart is a muscle and will actually gain in left ventricle wall thickness!) you will have to increase the rate at which you are moving to get up to a bpm that is optimal for fat burning. Remember, it's the bpm zone that is important in order to tap into the lipids (fat stores) that get released and used as fuel for your exercise bout.

Nutrition

Three major meals per day, snacks in between.

This is a very quick and general sample of what an approximate nutrition plan might look like. We won't get overcomplicated. You can use this as a guide for yourself. Or consult a qualified sports nutritionist if you want to get a more detailed plan.

Let's take a sample person and build a basic nutrition plan for them:

Alice is 55 years old, 165 pounds, with about 35% body fat. She wants to lose 25 pounds and has a normal range and variety of food she eats. No restrictions. We will assume she has a light resistance training routine two days per week, plus two days per week of cardio training.

We are going to determine her daily macros. These of course are *all* high-quality substrates—no fake foods. Earth foods only.

- Protein
- Carbohydrates
- Fats

For simplicity, here is what to do without getting super detailed:

Given that she has 35% body fat (most people are at least 25%, and it's not uncommon to be 40%), we can find her lean body mass (LBM) with this calculation:

$100\% - 35\% = 65\%$

165 lb. x 65% = 107 lb. LBM. This is approximate.

We are going to use her LBM for her daily protein intake in grams per day. This will change and be modified moving forward—it is just a starting point.

We will match her carbohydrate intake with 107 lb. LBM as well.

Alice's fat intake (again—good fats) will be 50% of 107.

Here's what it would look like:

PROTEIN 107 grams	=	428 calories
CARBS 107 grams	=	428 calories
FATS 53 grams	=	477 calories
Total base calories	=	1,333 daily
Snacking allowance additional		200–400 calories

This allows her up to approximately 1,733 daily calories with a minimum of 1,333 calories. This is very low but allows for snacking in between meals, which obviously increases calories. Protein target intake is *a must*.

Consume 100% of your complex carbohydrates (rice, pasta, potato) during the first two meals of the day (breakfast and lunch). I always allow snacking calories to meet the different daily fluctuations of hunger. The type of snacks is vitally important. I always recommend protein as a snack, then fruits and nuts—in that order. Never starve yourself. Keep the machine fed and blood sugar levels even—no spikes or dips.

This is the meal plan I would get Alice started on. We would tweak from here after six weeks. We want her in a slight caloric deficit because she wants to lose fat weight, starting with whole proteins, a daily must (yes, I said it twice). This is followed by dietary fat intake (good fats), then carbohydrates, which should be totally dominated by fruits and then veggies and complex carbs that, for this example, we've spread out between all three meals. Often, we will have our clients stop eating complex carbs at noon, thus eating only whole proteins and fruits and veggies at dinner.

If Alice gets inspired by the successful changes she starts to see, there is a really good chance she will want to up her game and really start to move the needle. This means increasing resistance training to three or even four days per week, along with her cardio sessions. This would mean increasing her macros. Specifically, her protein and carbohydrate intake would move up to around 125 grams per day to meet the demands of her increased training caloric burn and her increased recovery demands. This is growth. This is an anabolic lifestyle.

Example daily meal plan for Alice, based on the macros we calculated:

Daily Meal Plan: 1,333 Calories (approximately)

Macro Split: Approximately 35% Protein (116g), 35% Carbs (116g), 30% Fats (44g).

This meal plan ensures all protein comes from red meat, salmon, chicken, or eggs (all whole proteins!) with healthy fats and balanced carbs. Always leave a little wiggle room when making macro counts: +/− 3%–5%.

Breakfast: Egg and Salmon Scramble with Avocado

- Ingredients:
  - 3 large eggs (140 calories, 18g protein, 1g carbs, 10g fat)
  - 2 oz cooked salmon (110 calories, 14g protein, 0g carbs, 6g fat)
  - 1/2 oz avocado (25 calories, 1.5g carbs, 2.25g fat)
  - 1 slice whole-grain toast (80 calories, 4g protein, 15g carbs, 1g fat)
- Macros:
  - Calories: 355

- o Protein: 36g
- o Carbs: 17.5g
- o Fats: 19.25g

Lunch: Grilled Chicken with Quinoa and Olive Oil

- Ingredients:
  - o 4 oz grilled chicken breast (186 calories, 35g protein, 0g carbs, 4g fat)
  - o 1/3 cup cooked quinoa (73 calories, 2.5g protein, 13.5g carbs, 1.25g fat)
  - o 1 tbsp olive oil (120 calories, 0g protein, 0g carbs, 14g fat)
  - o 1 cup steamed broccoli (55 calories, 10g carbs, 0.5g fat)
- Macros:
  - o Calories: 434
  - o Protein: 37.5g
  - o Carbs: 23.5g
  - o Fats: 19.75g

Dinner: Lean Steak with Sweet Potato and Asparagus

- Ingredients:
  - o 5 oz lean sirloin steak (170 calories, 35g protein, 0g carbs, 7g fat)
  - o 1/2 medium sweet potato, baked (60 calories, 13g carbs, 0g fat)
  - o 1 cup steamed asparagus (27 calories, 5g carbs, 0g fat)
  - o 1 tsp grass-fed butter (35 calories, 0g protein, 0g carbs, 4g fat)
- Macros:
  - o Calories: 292
  - o Protein: 35g

- o Carbs: 18g
- o Fats: 11g

Approximate Daily Total:

- o Calories: 1,331
- o Protein: 116.25g (35%)
- o Carbs: 116g (35%)
- o Fats: 44g (30%)

This meal plan ensures all proteins are derived exclusively from whole proteins—red meat, salmon, chicken, and eggs (and quinoa, which is an exception)—and includes a balanced mix of carbs and healthy fats. Adjust portions slightly if needed to match your exact calorie and macro requirements.

REMEMBER: This is a low-caloric profile (Alice is in a calorie deficit here) that is enhanced by snacking allowance of up to approximately 400 additional calories (mostly snacks of protein and fats). For a person engaged in an adequate resistance and cardio schedule, these calorie allotments would all rise significantly and also change macro splits (% protein/carb/fats) during a macrocycle of training, depending on the targeted outcome. It is not uncommon to hit 2,500 to 3,500 calories on a daily basis when participating in the proper fitness program. Again, it depends on what the goal is.

So you want to shred fat off your body?

I have trained many athletes and competitive bodybuilders who have needed to cut weight or get super shredded for a competition—I mean in the 3% to 5% body fat shredded. It is actually mind blowing to see the human body become this defined. But remember, body fat percentage this low is unsustainable and not healthy, so *do not* get carried away.

If you are looking to really get aggressive and drop fat, not muscle, here is a 12 to 16 week protocol that I've used countless times to get my clients shredded.

1. Take the above diet example for Alice and cut out 80% of your complex carbs for eight to twelve weeks. I mean, literally 80% of your complex carbs (low amounts of rice, pasta, potato, oatmeal, or breads).

2. Eat whole proteins three to four times per day (heavy on red meat and whole eggs)—this time, 90% x your body weight to get your daily protein in grams), along with fresh whole fruits and veggies, and the good fats. Add in BCAA"s twice a day and our post workout 4:1 drink (in post-recovery section) is non-negotiable.

3. Add in about 30 grams of whole protein in the form of a protein shake *before* your cardio bouts. Do six days per week of cardio work (thirty minutes minimum) at the optimized bpm levels explained above and watch the fat fall off you.

4. Finally—keep your *proper* resistance training to at least two times per week during this 12-16 week period. It's not easy. You will run low on energy during these resistance bouts. You have to commit.

And remember—It's always better to have a base before you start something this aggressive. This means you should have had your baseline consistent workouts and nutritional routine going for at least three months ahead of a shredding program like this. You'll be more conditioned to handle the stress on your entire body and brain. And as always, there are modifications along the way to optimize this type of program.

CHAPTER 4

SUPPLEMENTATION

When you are placing above average or extreme demands on your system through proper fitness programming, your nutritional requirements increase in order to meet that demand. Supplements can be a terrific asset to assist in meeting the deficiencies that get created by high physical output. However, the supplement industry is rife with false claims and many scams. Here is a partial list of helpful rock-solid supplements that you can quickly source from Amazon. Remember, it's so easy to get carried away. I keep it simple and use foundational supplements to fortify my training and nutritional demand. So, keep it in check and use your earth food's nutrition to meet most of your requirements.

TWO INCREDIBLE WELLNESS/LONGEVITY HACKS

These are two tremendously beneficial daily hacks that are under $10 and are simple to incorporate.

Bio-Hack #1: Baking Soda in Water

How: Mix ½ to 1 teaspoon of baking soda (aluminum-free) into a glass of filtered water.

When: First thing in the morning or ninety minutes post-workout.

Science-Backed Benefits:

1. Reduces Acidity and Supports pH Balance – Helps buffer excess lactic acid, optimizing cellular function and reducing inflammation.
2. Boosts Athletic Performance – Acts as an ergogenic aid, delaying muscle fatigue by neutralizing acid buildup during intense workouts.
3. Aids Digestion – Helps with occasional heartburn or indigestion by neutralizing stomach acid naturally.
4. Supports Kidney Function – Shown to slow the progression of chronic kidney disease by reducing acid buildup in the blood.

Bio-Hack #2: Organic Apple Cider Vinegar (ACV)

How: Mix 1–2 tablespoons of organic ACV (not Bragg's—avoid due to "Apeel," a toxic chemical coating brought to you by Bill Gates) into 8 ounces of water.

When: Before meals or in the morning.

Science-Backed Benefits:

1. Stabilizes Blood Sugar – ACV improves insulin sensitivity and blunts post-meal glucose spikes.
2. Improves Digestion and Gut Health – ACV increases stomach acid and supports a healthy microbiome.
3. Supports Fat Metabolism – Shown to increase satiety and modestly reduce body fat over time.
4. Antimicrobial Properties – Naturally helps combat harmful bacteria and pathogens in the digestive tract.

These hacks cost pennies, require zero gym memberships, and can *immediately* support energy, performance, and resilience—especially when combined with a strong training protocol like The FITNESS QUADRANT.

GUT HEALTH:
THE POWER OF YOUR INTERNAL ECOSYSTEM

Before we venture into various supplements that can really assist you, let's first address the health of your stomach and digestive track ecosystem. This is a very important topic that can solve a myriad of issues you may be having both small and large. All the rights foods and supplements are far less effective if you stomach has issues and cannot process food intake effectively and efficiently so let's make sure it's strong and healthy first.

Your gut is home to trillions of bacteria that form a dynamic ecosystem called the microbiome. When balanced, these healthy bacteria aid digestion, support immune function, produce essential vitamins, regulate metabolism, and even influence mood and brain health. A diverse and abundant population of "good" bacteria acts as a protective barrier, keeping harmful microbes in check and maintaining overall vitality.

But when this balance is disrupted—through poor diet, stress, lack of sleep, overuse of antibiotics, and excessive alcohol or sugar intake— harmful bacteria can thrive. This leads to inflammation, weakened immunity, digestive problems, and an increased risk of chronic disease. In other words, the quality of your gut bacteria directly affects the quality of your health and longevity.

Habits That Damage Good Bacteria

- Antibiotic overuse – wipes out both harmful and beneficial bacteria.

- High sugar and processed food intake – fuels the growth of harmful bacteria and yeast.

- Excessive alcohol consumption – disrupts the microbiome balance.

- Chronic stress and lack of sleep – weakens the gut lining and reduces bacterial diversity.

- Artificial sweeteners and additives – shown in studies to negatively impact gut bacteria.

Top 5 Live Bacteria Food Sources

1. **Sauerkraut** – Fermented cabbage rich in probiotics and digestive enzymes.

2. **Greek Yogurt** – Contains live cultures that support gut flora and protein intake.

3. **Kefir** – A fermented milk drink with diverse strains of probiotics.

4. **Kimchi** – A spicy Korean fermented vegetable dish, loaded with beneficial bacteria.

5. **Kombucha** – A fermented tea beverage with probiotics and beneficial acids.

Be nice to your gut!

Gut Health: Good vs Bad Habits

✔ Eat fermented foods
(sauerkraut, yogurt, kefir, kimchi, kombucha)

✘ Overuse of antibiotics

✔ Consume fiber-rich foods
(fruits, vegetables, whole grains)

✘ High sugar & processed foods

✔ Get adequate sleep & reduce stress

✘ Excessive alcohol consumption

✔ Limit alcohol & sugar intake

✘ Chronic stress & lack of sleep

✔ Stay hydrated & active

✘ Artificial sweeteners & additives

WHEY PROTEIN

Biological value (BV) is a metric used to assess the *quality of a protein* by measuring the proportion of absorbed protein that is retained for bodily functions and growth. A higher BV indicates a protein source that closely matches the body's amino acid requirements, making it more efficient in supporting various physiological processes, including muscle building and repair.

BV is calculated by comparing the nitrogen content of absorbed protein to the nitrogen content of the protein retained. Nitrogen is a key component of amino acids, the building blocks of proteins.

The formula for BV is:

$$BV=(\text{Nitrogen absorbed}/\text{Nitrogen retained})\times 100$$

Here is a bar graph that measures and compares BV values:

Biological Value (BV) of Whole Proteins

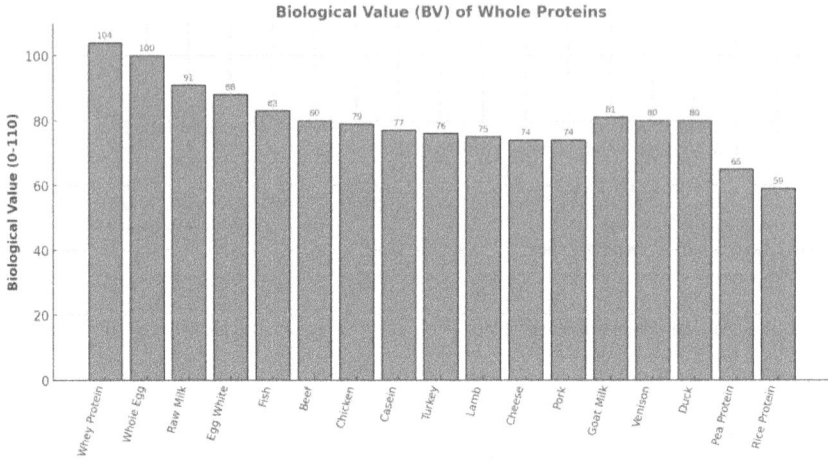

As you can clearly see, plant proteins are virtually half of the biological value as animal proteins. This is why nearly 99% of top athletes and successful fitness routines focus on high value animal proteins as the superior choice for nutritional values.

CREATINE

In addition to the profound and known physical benefits to muscle development and rapid energy supply, the May 2025 pilot trial in *Alzheimer's & Dementia: Translational Research & Clinical Interventions* (DOI 10.1002/trc2.70101), researchers Aaron N. Smith et al., based at the University of Kansas Medical Center presents promising early evidence that daily creatine (20g/day for eight weeks) significantly boosts brain creatine (~11%) and improves key memory and cognitive measures in Alzheimer's patients. This is the strongest human data so far supporting creatine as a supplement for memory support in neurodegenerative disease.

Creatine is one of the most studied and effective supplements on the market. Phosphagen creatine (PC), specifically creatine phosphate, plays a pivotal role as a major energy compound in the production of adenosine triphosphate (ATP) within the mitochondria. If you remember from previous chapters, ATP is often referred to as the "energy currency" of cells, and its availability is crucial for various cellular processes, particularly in the context of energy-demanding activities such as muscle contractions during fitness bouts.

Creatine phosphate, a high-energy compound stored in muscle cells, serves as a rapid and readily available reservoir of phosphate groups. When energy demand spikes, as is the case during intense physical activity (resistance training), the breakdown of ATP releases energy, leaving adenosine diphosphate (ADP) behind. Phosphagen creatine steps in by donating its phosphate group to ADP, converting it back into ATP.

This process is especially important during short bursts of high-intensity exercise, such as weightlifting or sprinting, where the demand for energy surpasses the immediate capacity of aerobic metabolism. The quick regeneration of ATP from ADP ensures that the muscle cells have a constant supply of energy to fuel contractions and maintain performance.

For athletes engaging in high-intensity and explosive activities, having adequate stores of phosphagen creatine is crucial for optimizing performance. Creatine is naturally found in small amounts in foods like meat and fish, and supplementation has become a common practice among athletes to enhance phosphagen creatine stores in muscles.

By increasing the availability of creatine phosphate, athletes can extend their capacity for short bursts of intense effort. This can lead to improvements in strength, power, and overall exercise performance. Additionally, enhanced ATP regeneration through creatine phosphate supports quicker recovery between bouts of high-intensity exercise.

While creatine phosphate primarily operates in the cytoplasm of cells, the mitochondria also play a vital role in ATP production. Mitochondria are the cellular organelles responsible for aerobic respiration, a process that yields a substantial amount of ATP. Although creatine phosphate is not directly involved in mitochondrial ATP synthesis, its role in the cytoplasm indirectly supports the energy needs of mitochondria by ensuring a constant supply of ATP during periods of increased demand.

Whether obtained through dietary sources or supplementation, creatine continues to be a valuable tool for athletes looking to maximize their energy reserves and achieve peak physical performance.

HYDRATION SUPPLEMENT

There are many hydration supplements on the market. Amazon offers a plethora. I like ones void of sweeteners, high in potassium and sea salt or Himalayan salt and extremely low in sugars. Hydration is essential for maintaining optimal physical and mental performance, as water supports nearly every bodily function, including temperature regulation, digestion, and nutrient transport. However, hydration isn't just about water—electrolytes, like sodium, potassium, magnesium, and calcium, are critical for cellular function, nerve signaling, and muscle contractions.

Quality electrolytes, such as those found in natural sources like pink Himalayan salt, provide trace minerals that enhance hydration by supporting electrolyte balance. Unlike processed table salt, pink Himalayan salt contains up to eighty-four trace minerals, including magnesium, calcium, and potassium, which help regulate blood pressure, maintain pH balance, and improve muscle and nerve function.

Every morning when I wake up, I drink a large glass of water with a pinch of pink Himalayan salt or sea salt. Consuming a high-sodium electrolyte drink first thing in the morning—before coffee or breakfast—is beneficial for several reasons:

1. **Rehydrates After Sleep:** Overnight, the body loses water and electrolytes through respiration and sweat. Starting your day with a high-sodium drink replenishes these losses.

2. **Boosts Energy:** Sodium helps activate the adrenal glands and supports blood flow, enhancing energy and mental clarity.

3. **Prepares the Digestive System:** Rehydrating with electrolytes kickstarts metabolic processes and prepares the digestive system for the day ahead.

4. **Balances Electrolytes:** Sodium supports water retention in cells, ensuring effective hydration throughout the body.

5. **Minimizes Coffee's Dehydrating Effects:** Drinking sodium-rich water before coffee offsets caffeine's mild diuretic effect, protecting against dehydration.

A morning ritual of drinking water mixed with pink Himalayan salt is a simple, effective way to restore hydration, replenish vital minerals, and optimize your body for the day.

NITRIC OXIDE

Nitric Oxide (NO) supplementation has garnered considerable attention in the realm of health and fitness due to its potential benefits on vascular function, exercise performance, and overall cardiovascular health. NO is a crucial signaling molecule that plays a pivotal role in regulating blood flow, blood pressure, and various physiological processes.

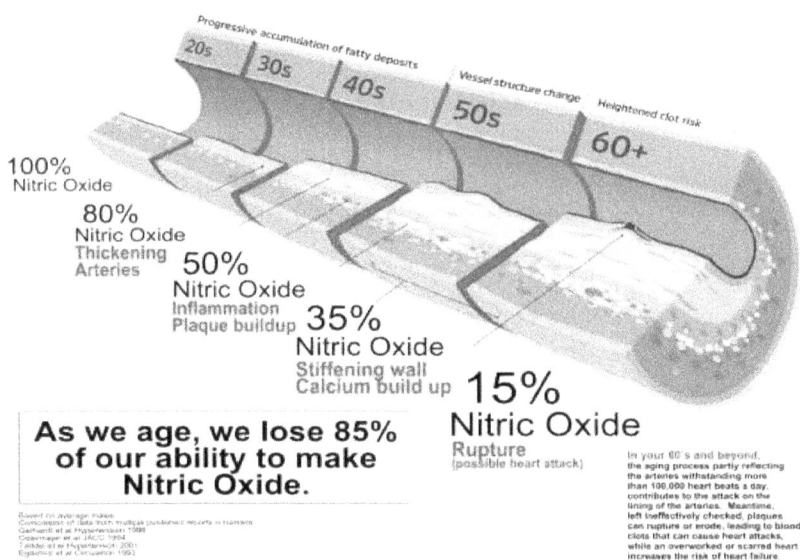

Progressive accumulation of fatty deposits

20s 30s 40s

Vessel structure change

50s

Heightened clot risk

60+

100% Nitric Oxide

80% Nitric Oxide
Thickening Arteries

50% Nitric Oxide
Inflammation Plaque buildup

35% Nitric Oxide
Stiffening wall Calcium build up

15% Nitric Oxide
Rupture (possible heart attack)

As we age, we lose 85% of our ability to make Nitric Oxide.

In your 60's and beyond, the aging process partly reflecting the arteries withstanding more than 100,000 heart beats a day, contributes to the attack on the lining of the arteries. Meantime, left ineffectively checked, plaques can rupture or erode, leading to blood clots that can cause heart attacks, while an overworked or scarred heart increases the risk of heart failure.

Based on average intake. Compilation of data from multiple published reports in numbers. Gerhardt et al Hypertension 1998. OppenHeimer et al JACC 1994. Taddel et al Hypertension 2001. Egashira et al Circulation 1993.

Benefits of Nitric Oxide Supplementation:

Improved Vasodilation: NO acts as a vasodilator, relaxing and widening blood vessels. This results in improved blood flow, which can have positive implications for cardiovascular health, exercise performance, and the delivery of oxygen and nutrients to tissues.

Enhanced Exercise Performance: Increased blood flow and oxygen delivery to muscles can contribute to improved exercise performance. Studies suggest that NO supplementation may lead to increased endurance, reduced fatigue, and better overall exercise efficiency.

Blood Pressure Regulation: NO helps regulate blood pressure by dilating blood vessels and promoting healthy endothelial function. Maintaining optimal NO levels may contribute to blood pressure homeostasis, reducing the risk of hypertension and related cardiovascular issues.

Anti-Inflammatory Effects: NO has anti-inflammatory properties, and its supplementation may have potential benefits in mitigating inflammation within the cardiovascular system and other tissues.

Numerous scientific studies have explored the effects of NO supplementation, revealing promising findings. Research has demonstrated that dietary sources of nitrates, which the body converts into NO, can positively impact cardiovascular health. Moreover, studies on specific NO precursor supplements, such as L-arginine and beetroot juice, have shown improvements in blood flow, exercise performance, and endothelial function.

As individuals age, there is a natural decline in NO production. Around the age of 50, NO levels may start to decrease, and by the time individuals reach 75, the decline becomes more rapid. This age-related reduction in NO has been associated with impaired vascular function, increased arterial stiffness, and a higher risk of cardiovascular diseases.

BCAAS: FUNCTION AND ROLE

Branched-chain amino acids (BCAAs) are essential amino acids with critical functions in protein synthesis, energy production, and muscle preservation. Athletes, especially those training for strength, muscle power, and growth, can benefit significantly from BCAA supplementation. By supporting muscle recovery, preventing breakdown, and enhancing protein synthesis, BCAAs play a crucial role in optimizing performance, reducing fatigue, and promoting overall muscle health for athletes pursuing their fitness goals.

Protein Synthesis: One of the primary functions of BCAAs, especially leucine, is to stimulate protein synthesis. Protein synthesis is the process by which the body builds new proteins, including muscle proteins. Leucine, in particular, activates the mTOR pathway, a key signaling pathway that regulates muscle protein synthesis.

Energy Source During Exercise: BCAAs can serve as an energy source during prolonged or intense physical activity. When the body's glucose stores become depleted, BCAAs can be broken down for energy, helping to sustain muscle function and prevent muscle breakdown, a process known as catabolism.

Muscle Preservation: BCAAs play a crucial role in preserving muscle mass, especially during periods of calorie restriction or intense training. By providing a direct source of energy and supporting protein synthesis, BCAAs contribute to the maintenance of lean muscle tissue.

Reducing Fatigue: Isoleucine and valine, two of the BCAAs, are involved in energy production and can help reduce exercise-induced fatigue. By competing with tryptophan, another amino acid that contributes to the perception of fatigue, BCAAs can delay the onset of exhaustion during prolonged exercise.

BCAAs are considered a critical supplement for athletes, particularly those training for strength, muscle power, and muscle growth, for several reasons:

Muscle Recovery: During intense resistance training, muscle fibers undergo microtears, and BCAAs play a key role in repairing and rebuilding these damaged tissues. Supplementing with BCAAs post-exercise can accelerate the recovery process, reducing muscle soreness and promoting faster healing.

Enhanced Protein Synthesis: Leucine, in particular, is a potent stimulator of muscle protein synthesis. Athletes aiming for muscle growth and strength can benefit from increased leucine levels, ensuring that their bodies have the necessary building blocks for optimal protein synthesis.

Preventing Muscle Breakdown: Athletes engaged in rigorous training, especially those in a calorie deficit, are at risk of muscle breakdown. BCAAs act as a buffer against catabolism by providing a direct source of energy and supporting protein synthesis, helping athletes maintain muscle mass even during challenging training phases.

Reducing Fatigue and Improving Endurance: By supplying energy during exercise and mitigating the perception of fatigue, BCAAs contribute to improved endurance. This is particularly valuable for athletes involved in high-intensity or prolonged activities.

GLUTAMINE

Glutamine is a conditionally essential amino acid that plays a multifaceted role in the human body, contributing to various physiological functions. While the body can synthesize glutamine to some extent, certain conditions, such as illness, stress, or intense physical activity, may increase the demand for this amino acid, making it essential in certain situations. While glutamine is not classified as an essential amino acid under normal circumstances, its importance becomes evident in specific contexts, including immune system function and the potential role it may play in avoiding colds.

Role of Glutamine:

> **Immune System Support:** Glutamine is a critical component of the immune system, playing a vital role in the function of immune cells. Immune cells, such as lymphocytes and macrophages, utilize it as a primary energy source. During times of increased immune activity, such as when the body is fighting off infections or dealing with stress, the demand for glutamine rises.

> **Cellular Energy Source:** Glutamine serves as a key substrate for cellular energy production, particularly in rapidly dividing cells like those of the immune system and the gastrointestinal tract. It participates in various metabolic pathways, including the tricarboxylic acid cycle, providing energy for cells and supporting their functions.

> **Gastrointestinal Health:** Glutamine plays a crucial role in maintaining the integrity of the gastrointestinal mucosa. It serves as fuel for the cells lining the digestive tract, promoting the health and function of the gut lining. This is particularly important for preventing leaky gut syndrome and supporting overall digestive health.

Glutamine and Avoiding Colds:

While glutamine's role in avoiding colds is not fully understood, some studies suggest a potential connection between glutamine supplementation and immune function. The logic behind this lies in the immune-boosting properties of glutamine. As a key player in immune cell function, it may contribute to a more robust defense against pathogens, including the viruses that cause the common cold.

During times of stress, illness, or intense physical activity, the body's glutamine stores may become depleted. This depletion could potentially compromise immune function, making individuals more susceptible to infections, including colds. By supplementing with glutamine, individuals may help support their immune system and reduce the risk of falling ill.

It's important to note that while there is some evidence suggesting a potential benefit of glutamine supplementation in certain situations, further research is needed to establish clear guidelines and confirm the extent of its impact on cold prevention. Additionally, individual responses to glutamine supplementation may vary, and it is always advisable to consult with a healthcare professional before incorporating any new supplement into your routine.

MULTI MINERAL AND VITAMIN

High-Quality multivitamin and mineral supplements play an important role in rigorous training.

The three I use year-round that are in addition to most of the above mentioned supps, are a longevity multivitamin combo with magnesium and a liquid ocean mineral supplement I drop into my water (or coconut water).

I use a brand of mineral and multivitamin supplements called PURE. You can get them on Amazon easily. I also use minor minerals supplementation that is derived from ocean minerals (sea salts) called ConcenTrace. Ocean minerals are some of the most potent and balanced microminerals you can find. They are 100% absorbed because they are in their natural form, not factory form. I simply put a few drops in my stainless-steel water bottle every day. Simple.

Remember, engaging in a rigorous resistance and cardio training routine places heightened demands on the body, particularly in terms of nutrient requirements. A high-quality multivitamin and mineral supplement can play a pivotal role in supporting performance, recovery, and overall well-being.

Key Benefits:

1. **Enhanced Energy Production**
   Intense exercise increases the demand for micronutrients involved in energy metabolism, such as B vitamins, magnesium, and iron. These nutrients help convert food into usable energy, ensuring sustained performance during training.

2. **Improved Recovery**
   Vitamins C and E, along with zinc and selenium, have antioxidant properties that combat exercise-induced oxidative stress. This reduces muscle damage and promotes faster recovery between workouts.

3. **Support for Muscle Function**
   Calcium, magnesium, and potassium are crucial for proper muscle contraction and relaxation. Adequate intake helps prevent cramps and supports optimal neuromuscular function.

4. **Strengthened Immune System**
   Rigorous exercise can temporarily suppress the immune system. Nutrients like vitamin C, vitamin D, and zinc enhance immunity, reducing susceptibility to illness and helping maintain consistency in training.

5. **Bone and Joint Health**
   Resistance training and high-impact cardio put stress on bones and joints. Vitamins D and K, along with magnesium and calcium, support bone density and joint integrity, reducing the risk of injury.

6. **Metabolic Health**
   A robust training regimen enhances metabolic activity, requiring sufficient levels of trace minerals like chromium, manganese, and iodine for hormonal balance and efficient metabolic process.

Why Quality Matters:

There is so much garbage out there in the supplement world. Just be careful and do your research. A high-quality supplement ensures optimal bioavailability, meaning the body can effectively absorb and utilize the nutrients. It also avoids fillers and subpar ingredients, providing a balanced spectrum of vitamins and minerals in their most active forms.

Incorporating a premium multivitamin and mineral supplement into a fitness-focused lifestyle acts as a safety net, bridging potential nutritional gaps and enabling the body to perform at its peak. For individuals pursuing ambitious fitness goals, it is a valuable investment in health and performance longevity.

POST-WORKOUT RECOVERY DRINK

This is perhaps one of the greatest opportunities to build muscle. It's one of the only times simple sugars (fruit juice) is a great asset to your body. Post-workout recovery is a segment of time that, if treated properly, is an enormous opportunity that is often ignored by the fitness community and certainly the mainstream segment of society that occasionally workout. After adequate resistance workouts, the body enters a catabolic state, characterized by muscle breakdown due to depleted glycogen stores and elevated cortisol levels. Consuming a high-quality post-workout recovery drink within the 45-minute window of opportunity is essential for transitioning from a catabolic to an anabolic state, where muscle repair and growth occur. Remember, a catabolic state means we are losing muscle, anabolic means we are building muscle. After the 45-minute window, it is very difficult to transition into an anabolic state from a supplemental drink. It now takes four to six hours to turn off the catabolic machine. I personally mix six ounces of pure grape juice or eight ounces of freshly made watermelon juice (one of my favorite go-to drinks—I make this all the time and keep it in my fridge) with one tablespoon of whey protein.

Key Benefits of 4:1 Mixture:

1. **Rapid Glycogen Replenishment**
   The simple carb-protein mix in a 4:1 ratio replenishes glycogen stores more efficiently than carbs alone, restoring energy levels and preparing muscles for future performance.

2. **Optimized Muscle Protein Synthesis**
   The inclusion of protein in the sugar mix stimulates muscle repair and growth by triggering insulin release from the sugar, thus creating a rapid increase of glucose uptake into the muscle and carrying the essential amino acids along with it, promoting an anabolic environment essential for recovery and muscle growth. Remember, amino acids are the building blocks of muscle!

3. **Reduced Muscle Damage and Fatigue**
   The formula contains antioxidants and other nutrients that combat oxidative stress, reducing post-workout inflammation and soreness for faster recovery.

4. **Improved Hormonal Balance**
   The carefully balanced carbs and protein help reduce cortisol levels while boosting insulin response, facilitating nutrient delivery to muscle cells for repair and growth.

5. **Proven Effectiveness**
   Studies have demonstrated that a 4:1 carbohydrate-to-protein ratio enhances recovery by 55% more than carbohydrate-only drinks and improves endurance in subsequent sessions by up to 29%.

The Transition from Catabolic to Anabolic

This unique formula addresses the critical post-workout recovery window, halting muscle breakdown and initiating muscle repair within minutes. By replenishing glycogen and triggering protein synthesis, it shifts the body into a state of anabolism, essential for building strength, increasing muscle mass, and improving performance.

This 4:1 ratio mix is not just a supplement; it is a scientifically validated tool for athletes and fitness enthusiasts aiming to maximize recovery, reduce downtime, and enhance results.

SKINNY JIMMY – PART 2

64-year-old male ectomorph

6'1" 149 lb. – borderline anorexic

Retired C-suite Insurance Executive – statistical analyst/strategist

Hardcore, lifelong fitness enthusiast

Major injuries – lower back, knees, shoulders

Nutrition – major caloric deficits and substrate imbalances

Strategy:

Jimmy needed a total reboot for every quadrant. That reboot, as always, really meant an education in fitness practices, wellness, and longevity strategies in all four quadrants. While he was well intentioned and extremely dedicated to working out, at age 64, he was rapidly moving in the wrong direction. This resulted in an accelerated loss of muscle mass, more frequent injuries, less energy, and confusing daily workouts that were very scattered and amorphous. This was exacerbated by poorly executed exercise form (biomechanics), inadequate nutrition, and virtually zero recovery time.

In reality, resetting somebody who has been "working out" in their own way for years is much harder than educating someone who has very little or no experience working out. The sad truth is that people get stuck in their ways, and they think that because they've been training for years, they have superior knowledge. The truth is, you can find some of the worst advice in the gym. The worst. This is simply one of many tragedies associated with the fitness industry.

DAY ONE

The very first thing I do with Jimmy, and everyone I work with, is meet for an hour to cover The FITNESS QUADRANT. It is the ultimate road map for anyone who is looking to embark on a true, scientifically based lifestyle. It identifies the four major phases of wellness, longevity, and fitness. You see, if one of the quadrants is missing or is being performed incorrectly, your journey will suffer greatly. Your expectations will never be met.

We start with how the pieces of the quadrants all fit together and are interconnected. How proper resistance training has to be met with adequate nutrition—the two-by-fours and nails of rebuilding muscle and meeting the energy needs of the human body. How cardiovascular work is vital to the respiratory system—heart and lungs. And finally, how recovery is a vital piece of the process.

Once this framework has been established, Jimmy and I get onto the gym floor and begin digging into exercise kinesiology and biomechanics. On day two—which is our first day actually performing exercises—we focus on resistance, the top left R in the quadrant. Jimmy is astonished. He finally understands how he has severely injured himself by performing exercises incorrectly, specifically his lower back, knees, and shoulders. This is the first light bulb that goes off in his head.

Jimmy asks, "How could I only exercise for 45 minutes using your system and get enough of a workout? I usually work out for ninety minutes."

"People fall into this trap where they think they have to spend hours in the gym to get significant reps, sets, etc." I reply. "There are very important triggers—hundreds of them—that dictate how the human musculature will respond to the signal of resistance and how it will adapt to that stimulus. It is about how many motor units you can fire on each rep and set, and whether or not you are leveraging ATP during the resistance exercise bout. This will determine whether the muscle will be triggered to adapt to the stress."

Jimmy asks, "Well, how many sets will we do in a 45-minute workout?"

I reply, "On average, we will perform 4 to 6 movements, in a certain pattern and sequence, that will fully leverage ATP, recruiting maximum motor units, and we will do 24–27 sets in 45 minutes"

Jimmy says, "What? It takes me 90 minutes to do 24 sets in my routine."

I reply, "Yes, I know. You, like millions of people that work out, don't understand bioenergetics and the power of the ATP-PC pathway and biomechanics, which are the focus of our modified interval training system. *You will work out half as long while you're at the gym and also cut your days working out in half, and you will get three times the success and results you've always wanted.* Welcome to The FITNESS QUADRANT and my MIT system."

SECTION 3 TAKEAWAYS

- Highly effective fitness is a combination of the four phases of fitness, R+N+C+R.

- Proper resistance training is the king of fitness modalities; it's where muscle is made.

- Proper nutrition, especially protein intake, is essential for building muscle mass.

- Adequate cardio work is essential for burning fat and maintaining a strong heart and lungs.

- Post-workout nutrition recovery is a vital part of switching into anabolic growth mode.

- Long-term recovery and social connectivity with true friends are vital to great physical and mental health.

- Mobility exercises are essential for moving freely and maintaining joint health.

- Sedentary and non-fitness people *especially* should incorporate baseline resistance exercises and then build up from there. Fitness has an entry point and place for everyone.

SECTION 4

THE FITNESS SCIENCE MATTERS

There are so many physical and neurological functions that get triggered and activated during a workout—whether it's a resistance session or a cardio bout—that to describe 10% of them would fill volumes of an encyclopedia series on its own. The information I've included below is a mere scratch of the surface—a small, selected handful of important and very interesting pieces that many people are unaware of. They usually react with spiked curiosity and heightened interest when they discover them. They all apply to our FITNESS QUADRANT and MIT system, and we actually refer to many of these scientific nuggets when we onboard and educate our clients. It typically drives new people to be much more dedicated to practice and develop a strategic game plan for choosing healthy and strong over sick and weak.

Remember, the human body is an amazing machine—the most intricate machine ever designed—and it is highly adaptive and responsive to the stimulus you feed it. Good stimulus drives anabolic growth, poor stimulus or a lack of stimulus drive catabolic decay and injury. This goes for both physical and mental stimuli. This is the part that is much bigger than just a workout at the gym. This is the 30,000-foot view looking down at what is actually happening when you turn on The FITNESS QUADRANT in your life. It's the ripple effect that radiates to everything and everyone around you. It's not just about achieving a more "in shape" or sculpted body or a lower bpm. It's about the good things that grow and become a part of you that you don't even realize, which make up your personal power and can help you push back against this harsh world. By turning on the quadrant, you become a better spouse, father or mother, brother or sister, daughter or son. A better friend, a better coach, a better businessperson, a better leader in your community. You set the pace by example and maybe make the world a little bit better, one rep at a time. Believe. It can happen to you.

CHAPTER 1

BODY COMPOSITION

Understanding the difference between lean body mass, which is comprised of mostly muscle weight, bone, and organs, and fat weight, that is primarily subcutaneous and visceral, is important to grasp. How they change in mass and size is vital to your journey.

When I hear unqualified fitness people talk about "weight loss," it drives my blood pressure to very high levels. There is good weight (muscle), and there is fat weight (mostly adipose tissue). Body fat percentage in amounts of 30% and more is not healthy. The first thing to understand is you do not want to lose muscle from your body. Ever. The more muscle you lose, your body fat percentage automatically increases without even gaining more body fat. As stated before, muscle is a major component related to your health status and a marker of longevity. Fat is what we are trying to lose and manage through proper fitness practices—*not* muscle. And how do we gain muscle? Adequate resistance training is the stand alone catalyst.

Here's an example: If you end up losing 30 pounds of "weight" on your "magic cleanse that my best friend Patty did," and 19 pounds of it was muscle, you are screwed at many levels. This is key to understanding the hows and whys of staying healthy and strong and not rotting into decay and weakness. The ability to lose fat and preserve muscle is science, plain and simple. You have to have the knowledge in order to do this.

Body composition, as opposed to just total body weight, is a critical measure of fitness and health. It provides a more comprehensive understanding of an individual's physical condition by breaking down the body into its different components, such as muscle, fat, bone, and other tissues. Nothing pisses me off more than witnessing products or celebrities that tout weight loss or diets as health remedies. It is totally misleading and most of them know it. Losing muscle along with fat as part of any weight loss program is not only harmful to your health but misguided and completely the opposite of what you're going to need to do if your goal is health and vitality.

On TV, you might have seen Marie Osmond as a spokesperson for Weight Watchers promoting huge health claims by guaranteeing 30 pounds of weight loss in 30 days or the ridiculous company Awaken 180° diet program claiming in past TV ads "you don't even need to work out to get healthy." Or how about ads for the supplement company, Balance of Nature, claiming miraculous health success eating little processed pills of powdered vegetables and fruits to lose "weight"—just sign up and eat their supplements and you'll lose all the weight you need and be healthy at last. These companies in my professional opinion are criminal, and they are spreading total lies to the unsuspecting public. It's a lie, and it's part of the problem of the current health crisis in the USA. Our national health is deteriorating at a more rapid pace thanks to the companies that push this garbage narrative.

Your goal is to lose fat weight and gain muscle weight. So, in turn, you need to gain weight (muscle!) in order to lose weight (fat!). It is important to realize that muscle is a major metabolic engine that will torch calories off your body—calories mostly in the form of fat, if you get your nutrition right. This is a critical piece of the puzzle that most people do not understand.

Here's a detailed summary of why body composition is a more meaningful measure of fitness than weight and of the role of muscle in this context:

Distinguishing Between Muscle and Fat: Total body weight alone does not differentiate between muscle mass and fat mass. This is crucial, because these two components have vastly different implications for overall health. Muscle is a metabolically active tissue that burns calories even at rest, while excess body fat, which burns zero calories, is associated with various health risks, including heart disease, diabetes, and more. Understanding the ratio of muscle to fat is, therefore, far more informative than knowing only your weight.

Muscle's Metabolic Benefits: Muscle is a metabolically active tissue, and the more muscle you have, the higher your RMR. This means that individuals with more muscle burn more calories even when they're at rest. Therefore, muscle mass contributes to an increased ability to manage body weight and maintain a healthier metabolism. Furthermore, it is associated with better insulin sensitivity, improved glucose control, and a reduced risk of metabolic diseases.

Role of Resistance Training: To increase muscle mass, sufficient resistance training, also known as strength or weight training, is essential. When resistance training is coupled with an appropriate diet, muscle development occurs.

Adaptive Mechanisms in Hypertrophy: The process of muscle hypertrophy involves several adaptive mechanisms. During resistance training, muscles are subjected to mechanical stress, leading to microscopic damage. In response, the body adapts by repairing and enlarging the muscle fibers. This growth is mediated by various factors, including the release of growth-promoting hormones like testosterone, IL-10, BDNF, and insulin-like growth factor (IGF-1), to name a few.

Body Composition and Health: Beyond aesthetics and athletic performance, body composition has profound implications for health. A lower body fat percentage and a higher muscle-to-fat ratio are associated with a reduced risk of chronic diseases, improved cardiovascular health, and better overall metabolic function. Conversely, an excess of body fat, particularly visceral fat (fat stored around the internal organs), is linked to inflammation and a range of metabolic disorders.

Functional Fitness: Functional fitness is a term that is defined as performing specific exercises that mimic everyday movement patterns and firing chains (several muscles that are linked together in a bodily movement)—or sport-specific exercises and movements and firing chains. These exercises improve your ability to function with greater strength and with less effort through normal daily movements or specific athletic movements. Having a higher percentage of muscle and proprioception (muscle memory) means greater strength, endurance, balance, recovery/reaction time, and mobility. It enhances an individual's ability to perform everyday activities, sport-specific movements, and also greatly reduces the risk of injuries like slip and falls, which are a major risk factor for people 65 years and older. Functional fitness relates to body composition in that a higher percentage of muscle is usually commensurate with an increase of functional capacity.

Understanding body composition is far more meaningful than just considering total body weight. The importance of muscle, and the fact that it can only be gained through resistance training, underscores the significance of a well-balanced fitness regimen that incorporates strength training. Focusing on optimizing body composition, with an emphasis on increasing muscle and reducing excess body fat, will lead to better overall health, improved metabolic function, and a higher quality of life. It's essential for individuals to prioritize both health and, for certain people, desired aesthetics by embracing a legitimate approach to fitness that includes resistance training as a primary fundamental component.

CHAPTER 2

GENETIC SOMATOTYPE

Somatotype is a classification system developed by psychologist William Sheldon in the 1940s to describe an individual's natural body type and physical characteristics. It is based on genetic predisposition, body composition, and metabolic tendencies. While the system is somewhat simplified, it provides a useful framework for understanding how different people respond to diet, exercise, and lifestyle changes.

THE THREE SOMATOTYPES

1. **Ectomorph** – Very thin, narrow type body

   Physical Traits: Slim, lean, and often tall with narrow shoulders and hips.

   Metabolism: Naturally high metabolic rate, making it harder to gain weight.

   Tendencies:

   > Weight Loss: Prone to losing weight easily.
   > Muscle Gain: Struggles to build muscle mass or retain fat.

2. **Mesomorph** – Relatively medium size, V-shaped torso

   Physical Traits: Athletic and muscular build with a naturally higher proportion of muscle mass and a medium frame.

   Metabolism: Efficient metabolism; can easily adapt to weight loss or gain.

Tendencies:

Weight Loss/Gain: Can lose or gain weight with relative ease, depending on diet and activity.
Muscle Gain: Naturally predisposed to gaining muscle.

3. **Endomorph** – Wide hips, narrow shoulders, pear-shaped

Physical Traits: Rounder or softer body shape with a higher percentage of body fat and a wider frame.

Metabolism: Slower metabolic rate, making it easier to gain weight and harder to lose it.

Tendencies:

Weight Gain: Susceptible to gaining fat quickly, especially with excess caloric intake.
Weight Loss: Requires more effort and consistency to lose weight.

Summary:

- **Ectomorphs:** Need to focus on caloric surplus and strength training to gain weight or muscle.

- **Mesomorphs:** Thrive on balanced nutrition and can adapt to various fitness goals with ease.

- **Endomorphs:** Benefit from a disciplined approach to diet and exercise, prioritizing activities that boost metabolism and promote fat loss.

Understanding somatotypes can help tailor fitness and nutrition strategies to maximize results, but it's important to remember that most people are a combination of these types rather than fitting perfectly into one category. We have trained several hundred people over the years, and as you can imagine, we have seen a large variation in all these types. I strongly believe the onboarding of anyone new who has goals that are inconsistent with the reality of what they are shooting for is a major issue that needs to be professionally addressed with them.

One of the most misleading components of the fitness industry is people selling the dream of looking like some genetic freak on a magazine cover. A 6'4" handsome male, 235 pounds of muscle, 8% body fat, tan and tatted, shredded V-shaped body, with thighs like ripped tree trunks. Or that gorgeous 5'10" female bombshell with long thick hair, long muscular legs and glutes—I'll stop there—who is gracing the cover of every sports publication and social media channel on earth. If an endomorph who is 90 pounds overweight comes in wanting to look like that guy on the magazine or that model girl, I make a point of getting them to shift their focus onto themselves and forget about other people's looks. Yes, it's inspiring, and it's eye candy, but in most cases it's extremely misleading. Fitness and wellness are much bigger, more rewarding, and deeper than glamorous vanity, which most of the time is empty and short-lived. We all age, and we all lose that youthful look sooner or later. Training for quality and longevity of life is attainable for everyone. Train for the right reasons, no matter your looks.

CHAPTER 3

CENTRAL NERVOUS SYSTEM

YOU ARE 100,000 MILES OF CIRCUITRY

The human nervous system is astonishingly vast and complex. Scientists estimate that the average adult brain contains about 86 billion neurons, each forming thousands of connections (synapses) with others. If you added up the length of all the axons (the long, threadlike fibers that carry electrical signals between neurons), the total "wiring" of the human brain alone would stretch roughly 85,000 to 100,000 miles— about four times around the Earth. When you include the peripheral nervous system that extends throughout the body, the total neurological circuitry is thought to exceed 100,000 miles. This is MINDBLOWING!

Length of Human Neurological Circuitry vs. Earth's Circumference

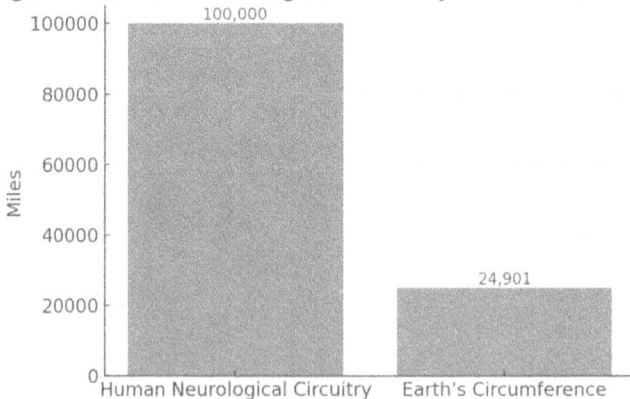

For someone who is new to resistance training and is coming off a sedentary lifestyle, or even for someone who isn't sedentary but just doesn't strength train, the first couple of months actually involve waking up your central nervous system (CNS). This is where the initial strength gains originate from. It's the CNS that learns how to recruit more muscle fiber during exercise. Only after this happens does the muscle starts to add little contractile proteins (actin and myosin) and grow. This is when you'll be able to start to see the first visible results of your efforts. For this exact reason, I tell people that proper fitness training and protocols take a little time to take root. You have to have an incremental mentality. It's not going to happen overnight. Anyone preaching that crap through social media ads is lying. This misleading advice is another example of what is wrong with the fitness industry, in my very experienced opinion. Unrealistic fitness expectations have brought a quitting mentality to millions of people because they don't see any progress in the first twelve days. What a shame.

The human body possesses an intricate network of neurological pathways and nerves that play a crucial role in maintaining overall health, well-being, and fitness capabilities. This complex system allows for effective communication between the brain, spinal cord, and the rest of the body. There is no better way to enhance and strengthen the CNS than resistance training.

Neurological pathways refer to the connections formed by neurons, which are specialized cells responsible for transmitting electrical signals throughout the body. These pathways enable the brain to receive and interpret sensory information, initiate appropriate motor responses, and regulate various bodily functions. The nerve network, composed of peripheral nerves, connects the CNS (comprised of the brain and spinal cord) to the body's muscles, organs, and sensory receptors. These nerves carry signals back and forth, allowing for voluntary movement, involuntary actions, and the perception of sensations. The length of the nerve network as you see is vast, and it's extensive reach ensures that signals can be transmitted to every part of the body, enabling coordinated movements, reflexes, and sensory experiences.

The importance of a healthy neurological system cannot be overstated for overall health and well-being. It enables us to perform daily activities, engage in physical exercise, and respond to our environment effectively. When the neurological pathways and nerve network are functioning optimally, they facilitate smooth and efficient movement, aid in maintaining balance, and contribute to overall physical fitness.

Proprioception, or the body's ability to sense its position, movement, and force exertion, plays a vital role in functional movement patterns. It relies on specialized receptors called proprioceptors, which are located in muscles, tendons, and joints. These proprioceptors send constant feedback to the brain, providing information about limb position, muscle length and tension, and joint angles. By integrating proprioceptive feedback, the brain can accurately coordinate and control movement patterns. This is essential for activities such as walking, running, lifting objects, and maintaining proper posture. Proprioception helps prevent injuries by providing real-time information about body position and alignment, allowing for quick adjustments and adaptations during movement.

The CNS plays a crucial role in weight training. It is responsible for sending signals from the brain to the muscles, allowing them to contract and produce movement. When weight training, the CNS must work to recruit and activate the correct muscle fibers in order to perform the exercise correctly and with proper form. This recruitment and activation process is known as neuromuscular activation. Additionally, the CNS plays a role in adapting to the demands of weight training by increasing the number of muscle fibers that are recruited over time, leading to increased strength, muscle mass, and a major increase in the CNS neuromuscular activation, which means the body adapts by stimulating more muscle fiber (actin and myosin) to produce more strength by way of increased motor unit recruitment. Brilliant design!

Resistance Training and a Healthy CNS:

Resistance training, also known as strength or weight training, is a fundamental component of maintaining a healthy and vibrant CNS. The benefits of resistance training extend beyond muscle strength and encompass crucial aspects related to the CNS and its role in preventing slip and fall injuries.

1. **CNS Structure and Function:** The CNS integrates and processes information from the body and the external environment. The brain is the central control center responsible for cognitive functions, sensory perception, decision-making, and initiating motor actions. The spinal cord serves as a relay between the brain and the rest of the body, facilitating communication and controlling motor functions.

2. **Muscle Strength and Stability:** Resistance training helps in building muscle strength and enhancing muscle mass. Muscles act as crucial stabilizers, especially around joints and in weight-bearing activities. A strong musculature supports stability and balance, providing a protective mechanism against slips and falls.

4. **Neuromuscular Coordination:** Resistance training engages the CNS, improving neuromuscular coordination. The CNS learns to efficiently recruit muscle fibers for specific movements, enhancing control and balance. This heightened coordination is vital in reacting swiftly to sudden slips or imbalance, reducing the likelihood of falling.

5. **Muscle Motor Unit Firing:** Muscle motor units are fundamental components of muscle function. A motor unit consists of a motor neuron and the muscle fibers it innervates. Motor neurons in the spinal cord send electrical signals to muscle fibers, causing them to contract. The CNS regulates the firing of these motor units, determining the force and pattern of muscle contractions needed for specific movements.

7. **Bone Density and Joint Health:** Resistance training stimulates bone density and strengthens connective tissues around joints. Stronger bones and resilient joints are essential in maintaining stability and preventing fractures or injuries that can occur during a fall. This process starts with the CNS being stimulated to trigger voluntary muscle contractions.

8. **Proprioception:** Proprioception is the body's ability to sense its position, movement, and orientation in space. It relies on sensory feedback from proprioceptors (specialized nerve endings in muscles, tendons, and joints) that detect changes in muscle length, tension, and joint angle. This information is sent to the CNS, providing a sense of body position and movement, enabling coordinated and precise motor responses.

9. **Enhanced Proprioception:** Regular resistance training enhances proprioception. This heightened awareness of one's body and surroundings enables quicker and more accurate adjustments to prevent falls and maintain stability.

10. **Science of Proprioception for Stability and Athletic Performance:** Athletes benefit from enhanced proprioceptive abilities, which enable improved coordination, agility, and skill execution. Proprioceptive training helps athletes optimize muscle motor unit firing and refine movements, ultimately enhancing athletic performance and reducing the risk of injuries.

11. **Fall Prevention and Injury Mitigation:** With a stronger CNS and improved muscle strength and coordination, individuals are better equipped to respond effectively to situations that might cause slips or falls. The CNS, when trained through resistance exercises, aids in rapidly activating muscles to counterbalance and prevent a fall, reducing the risk of injury.

13. **Human Longevity and Well-being:** A well-functioning CNS is vital for longevity and overall well-being. Proper muscle motor unit firing and enhanced proprioception contribute to efficient movement, reducing the risk of falls and injuries, especially in the elderly. Engaging in physical and mental activities that challenge and stimulate the CNS can support its health, promoting a higher quality of life as individuals age.

The CNS, consisting of the brain and spinal cord, plays a central role in regulating muscle motor unit firing and proprioception, vital for movement, stability, and athletic performance. Understanding and optimizing proprioception through training can enhance performance and reduce injury risks. Maintaining a healthy CNS is essential for longevity and overall well-being throughout one's life.

Incorporating resistance training into a regular fitness routine contributes to long-term well-being. As people age, maintaining muscle strength and CNS function becomes increasingly crucial to prevent falls and fractures that can significantly impact overall health and quality of life.

Resistance training is pivotal for a healthy CNS, promoting muscle strength, neuromuscular coordination, bone density, and joint health. These benefits collectively contribute to enhanced stability and balance, guarding against slip and fall injuries. By maintaining a robust CNS through resistance training, individuals can lead an active and fulfilling life while minimizing the risks associated with accidents and falls.

The CNS is a highly intricate and crucial network within the human body, composed of the brain and spinal cord. Its function is paramount for various physiological processes, including muscle motor unit firing and proprioception, which are essential for movement, stability, athletic performance, and overall well-being.

NEUROGENESIS AND YOUR BRAIN HEALTH

Neurogenesis is the process of generating new neurons (nerve cells) in the brain, particularly in the hippocampus and certain other brain regions. This process is vital for learning, memory, and overall brain health. It was once believed that neurogenesis primarily occurred during development and was limited in adults, but we now know that it can occur throughout adulthood and is influenced by various factors, including physical exercise.

As you know by now, resistance exercise, or weight training, involves working against resistance to build muscle strength and endurance. It has been shown to stimulate neurogenesis and promote brain health, especially in the aging population. Here's how resistance exercise influences neurogenesis and its potential impact on delaying Alzheimer's disease:

1. **Stimulation of Growth Factors:** MIT Resistance exercise triggers the release of several growth factors that are essential for neurogenesis and brain health. These growth factors include:

   - Brain-Derived Neurotrophic Factor (BDNF): BDNF is a protein that promotes the growth, survival, and differentiation of neurons. It plays a crucial role in synaptic plasticity, which is essential for learning and memory.

   - Insulin-like Growth Factor-1 (IGF-1): IGF-1 is another growth factor that supports the growth and development of neurons and enhances synaptic plasticity.

   - Interleukin 10 (IL-10): A growth factor that is only released into the bloodstream when certain adequate resistance and cardiovascular stress is placed on the body. IL-10 shuts down interleukin 6 (IL-6), which is an inflammation hormone that is constantly in our system at low levels. This is why legitimate fitness protocols are central to triggering anabolic growth, thus turning the clocks back and reversing the catabolic aging (decay) process.

2. **Reduced Inflammation and Oxidative Stress:** Resistance exercise can reduce chronic inflammation and oxidative stress, which are factors associated with neurodegenerative diseases like Alzheimer's. Chronic inflammation and oxidative stress can damage neurons and impair neurogenesis. By decreasing these harmful processes, resistance exercise helps maintain a healthier brain environment.

3. **Increased Blood Flow to the Brain:** Resistance training improves cardiovascular health and increases blood flow to the brain. This enhanced blood flow delivers oxygen and nutrients to brain cells, supporting their function and viability. Improved circulation can also help in reducing the risk of cognitive decline and Alzheimer's disease.

4. **Improvement in Insulin Sensitivity:** Resistance exercise can enhance insulin sensitivity, which is crucial for brain health. Insulin resistance is linked to cognitive decline and Alzheimer's disease. By improving insulin sensitivity, resistance exercise may reduce the risk of developing these conditions.

5. **Beneficial Effects on Hormones:** Resistance exercise influences the release of hormones like cortisol and testosterone. Cortisol, when chronically elevated, can have detrimental effects on brain health, including impairing neurogenesis. On the other hand, testosterone has neuroprotective effects and can support neurogenesis.

For the aging population, these effects of resistance exercise on neurogenesis and brain health are particularly crucial. Aging is often associated with a decline in neurogenesis and an increased risk of cognitive decline, including Alzheimer's disease. Engaging in regular resistance exercise can help mitigate these age-related changes, enhance brain function, improve cognitive abilities, and potentially delay the onset and progression of Alzheimer's disease.

Plain and simple—resistance exercise promotes neurogenesis by stimulating growth factors, reducing inflammation and oxidative stress, enhancing blood flow to the brain, improving insulin sensitivity, and positively affecting hormones. These mechanisms are vital for brain health and are especially important for the aging population in reducing the risk of Alzheimer's disease and maintaining cognitive function. It is the very best medicine for longevity and quality of life.

Various studies on how strength training fights dementia and Alzheimer's disease:

Resistance training has been shown to have beneficial effects on cognitive function and brain health. Recent research suggests that weight training may help fight dementia and Alzheimer's disease by promoting neurogenesis, the growth of new nerve cells in the brain.

One study found that older adults who engaged in weight training twice a week for six months had an increase in the volume of the hippocampus, a brain region that is important for memory and spatial navigation. This increase in volume was associated with improved cognitive function, including memory and attention.

Another study found that weight training increased levels of BDNF, a protein that plays a role in the growth and survival of nerve cells. This suggests that weight training may promote neurogenesis in the brain, which could help protect against cognitive decline.

Weight training has also been found to improve blood flow to the brain, which can help nourish and protect brain cells. Additionally, weight training has been shown to have anti-inflammatory effects, which may also help protect the brain from damage.

Overall, the current research suggests that weight training can have a positive impact on cognitive function and brain health and may help protect against dementia and Alzheimer's disease by promoting neurogenesis in the brain. However, more research is needed to understand the full extent of the benefits of weight training for brain health and to determine the optimal type and frequency of weight training for different population groups.

Six research papers on top benefits of fitness training for Alzheimer's:

1. "Exercise and the Prevention of Alzheimer's Disease" by R.N. Cotman and N.C. Berchtold in *Trends in Neurosciences*. (2002)

2. "Physical Activity and Risk of Cognitive Decline and Dementia in Elderly Persons" by K.E. Laurin, et al. in *Archives of Neurology*. (2001)

3. "Physical Exercise and the Adult Brain: A Review of Proven Benefits" by J.F. Sabelhaus and D.A. Spirduso in *Journal of Aging and Physical Activity*. (2015)

4. "Physical Activity, Brain Plasticity and Alzheimer's Disease" by G. Cotman and N. Berchtold in *Current Opinion in Psychiatry*. (2002)

5. "Physical Activity and Dementia Risk: The FINGER Study" by T. Rantanen, et al. in *JAMA Neurology*. (2015)

6. "The Role of Aerobic Fitness in Cognitive and Brain Health: The Current State of the Evidence" by A.L. McMorris, et al. in *Progress in Brain Research*. (2016)

CHAPTER 4

INSULIN FUNCTION

WHAT IS INSULIN AND HOW DOES IT WORK?

Insulin is a hormone that plays a vital role in managing your body's energy. It's produced by your pancreas and works like a key, unlocking your cells to allow glucose (sugar) to enter and provide energy. Without insulin, your cells wouldn't be able to absorb the glucose from the foods you eat, and your body would struggle to use food as fuel properly.

When you eat, especially foods with carbohydrates, they break down into glucose, which enters your bloodstream. This triggers your pancreas to release insulin. Insulin then helps your cells absorb glucose to either use immediately for energy or store it as glycogen in your muscles and liver for later. This process is essential for maintaining balanced blood sugar levels and giving your body the energy it needs to function.

INSULIN HEALTH VERSUS INSULIN RESISTANCE

Insulin health refers to the proper functioning of insulin in the body. When your insulin sensitivity is high, your cells respond efficiently to insulin, allowing glucose to enter your cells with ease. This means your body can effectively manage blood sugar levels, use energy efficiently, and avoid energy crashes. Healthy insulin levels also help in muscle growth because the hormone promotes nutrient uptake into cells, including amino acids (the building blocks of muscle) and glucose, which are vital for muscle repair and growth.

Insulin resistance, on the other hand, is when your body's cells stop responding well to insulin. It's like your cells become numb to the signal insulin is trying to send, so the glucose doesn't get absorbed effectively. As a result, your pancreas compensates by producing more insulin to try to push the glucose into the cells. Over time, this constant overproduction of insulin can lead to higher-than-normal blood insulin levels—a state called hyperinsulinemia.

When insulin resistance sets in, the body struggles to manage blood sugar, leading to higher glucose levels in the blood. This is a hallmark of type 2 diabetes but can also lead to other metabolic issues like obesity, inflammation, and heart disease. More importantly, it interferes with muscle growth because your body is less efficient at delivering nutrients like glucose and amino acids to muscle cells.

HOW INSULIN AFFECTS MUSCLE GROWTH

Insulin is actually an anabolic hormone, meaning it helps build and store things in the body, including muscle. After resistance training, your muscles need nutrients to repair and grow stronger. Insulin helps by delivering glucose (which fuels muscle cells) and amino acids (which are used to build muscle tissue) to the muscles. In this way, insulin helps muscle growth by increasing the availability of nutrients that are critical for recovery and muscle development.

When insulin is working well, your body has a better chance of utilizing these nutrients effectively, helping you recover faster and build more muscle over time. However, in a state of insulin resistance, your body can't use those nutrients as effectively, which hinders muscle recovery and growth.

INSULIN RESISTANCE AND METABOLIC DAMAGE

Metabolic damage refers to a breakdown in your body's ability to regulate basic functions like metabolism, hormone production, and energy balance. It's often the result of chronic poor diet, lack of exercise, and poor lifestyle habits. The main consequence of metabolic damage is that it disrupts the body's ability to burn fat and build muscle.

Insulin resistance is a significant part of this metabolic damage. When your cells become resistant to insulin, your body enters a state where it's constantly struggling to maintain healthy blood sugar levels. This leads to chronically high insulin levels in your bloodstream (because your pancreas is working overtime to compensate), and this elevated insulin state has several negative consequences:

Fat Storage: High insulin levels can promote fat storage, especially in the abdominal area, because insulin is a fat-storage hormone. The more insulin circulating, the more likely your body is to store fat, particularly if you're not using it for energy through physical activity.

Impaired Muscle Growth: As mentioned earlier, insulin is needed for muscle growth. But when insulin resistance occurs, your muscles don't get the nutrients they need, slowing down muscle repair and growth.

Chronic Inflammation: Insulin resistance is associated with higher levels of inflammation in the body, which can further disrupt metabolic processes, damage tissue, and promote disease.

Increased Risk of Disease: High insulin levels and insulin resistance are linked to several diseases, including type 2 diabetes, heart disease, and even certain cancers.

WHAT CAUSES INSULIN RESISTANCE?

Here are the four dark horsemen rearing their toxic heads again. Certain lifestyle factors can contribute to the development of insulin resistance and metabolic damage. Some of the key factors include:

Seed Oils: These are highly processed oils (like soybean, canola, and sunflower oil) that are common in many processed foods. They are high in omega-6 fatty acids, which, when consumed in excess, can cause inflammation in the body and contribute to insulin resistance.

Artificial Sweeteners: While they don't contain sugar, some studies suggest that artificial sweeteners can interfere with insulin response by changing the way your body processes sugar. This can increase insulin resistance over time.

Trans Fats: These are harmful fats found in many processed foods like fast food, baked goods, and snacks. Trans fats are associated with inflammation and insulin resistance, which can lead to metabolic damage.

Excessive Sugar and Refined Carbs: A diet high in sugar and refined carbohydrates (like white bread and pastries) can cause a spike in blood glucose levels, forcing your pancreas to release large amounts of insulin. Over time, this can exhaust your pancreas and make your cells resistant to insulin.

HYPER FAT STORAGE MODE

When you slam your body with sugar-packed foods like soda, fruit juice, candy bars, frosted cereals, fast carbs (see glycemic index pp 112) or so-called "healthy" snacks like sugar-loaded "energy" bars like Kind bars or Cliff bars, your blood sugar rockets up.

This spike triggers a surge of insulin—your body's fat-storage hormone—shoving excess sugar into fat cells.

At the peak of these spikes, fat storage goes into overdrive. Then comes the crash: insulin stays elevated, blood sugar drops, and you're left tired, foggy, and craving more sugar. Every spike-and-crash cycle multiplies fat gain and wrecks your energy all day long.

I made the following chart to illustrate this roller coaster ride. If you look at stabilized blood sugar levels in the middle where I point out Life Strong Zone—this is where learning how to select proper slow burning carbs or low glycemic index carbohydrates and stay far away from sugary high glycemic food items, will help you immensely in your battle to lose fat by staying out of the fat gaining zone. This is one of the many reasons our nutrition guidelines (and my personal lifestyle) leans heavily on consuming whole proteins and good fats as the priority.

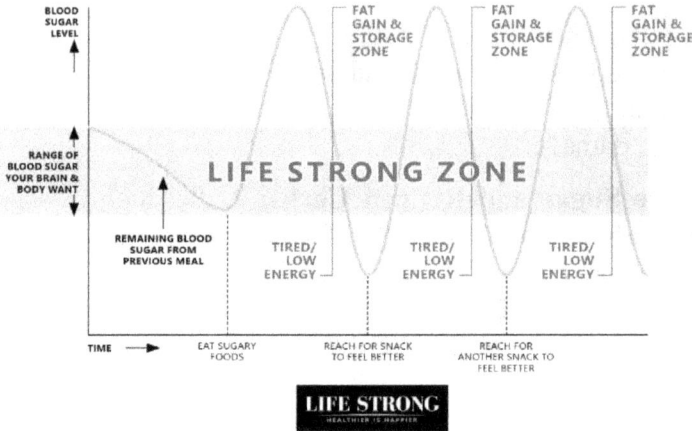

THE BOTTOM LINE

Insulin plays a crucial role in managing your body's energy, helping you grow muscle, and keeping your metabolism in check. Healthy insulin function supports muscle growth, fat loss, and overall energy balance. But when you become insulin resistant—due to poor lifestyle choices, including eating processed foods, seed oils, fake sugars, and trans fats—your body's ability to manage blood sugar and support muscle growth is compromised.

Insulin resistance is a sign of metabolic damage, which is a major risk factor for chronic diseases like type 2 diabetes and cardiovascular disease. To support your body's insulin health, it's important to focus on a whole-foods-based diet, regular exercise, and avoiding the processed foods that contribute to metabolic damage.

CHAPTER 5

INSIDE THE FITNESS MATRIX

As you dive into The FITNESS QUADRANT, you're not just exercising, you're unleashing the science—you're unlocking a series of powerful internal processes that transform your body and health with every workout, every rep, and every drop of sweat. You will not only look different and become totally in shape over time, but you'll also become an example for everyone in your network, especially your spouse and kids. What better gift to give them than the gift of healthy and strong!

When you grasp the deeper science behind what you're doing, it changes everything. Understanding the *why* behind your training fuels your drive, making you more committed and consistent. The internal fitness matrix is massive and virtually never ending, and it's all linked together. Amazing!

Out of the hundreds of biological and chemical processes, here are a handful I selected that aren't just fascinating, they're keys to a whole new level of vitality. These are the unseen functions to the biology and science that keep you strong, youthful, and unstoppable.

UNLOCKING YOUR BODY'S INTERNAL HIDDEN POWERS WITH THE FITNESS QUADRANT

SYNOVIAL FLUID

Time to lube yourself up. Synovial fluid is a crucial component of synovial joints, which include the majority of joints in the human body. Its importance lies in its ability to lubricate and nourish the joints, ensuring smooth movement and reducing friction during articulation. The synovial fluid acts as a shock absorber, distributing pressure evenly within the joint and providing stability. Moreover, it assists in nutrient and waste exchange between the cartilage and surrounding blood vessels.

As we age, the production of synovial fluid decreases, and its quality may diminish. This reduction in production is partly due to a decrease in the cells responsible for synthesizing the fluid, such as synoviocytes, as well as changes in the composition of the fluid itself. This can lead to joint stiffness, decreased range of motion, and an increased risk of joint-related issues like osteoarthritis.

Resistance training plays a significant role in enhancing the body's ability to produce robust amounts of synovial fluid. When engaging in resistance exercises, the joints experience controlled stress and loading, stimulating the production of synovial fluid to facilitate smooth movement and protect the joint surfaces. The mechanical compression and decompression during these exercises encourage the synoviocytes to produce and maintain a healthy volume of synovial fluid, promoting joint health and mobility.

Weight training can increase synovial fluid in joints, leading to improved flexibility. Synovial fluid is produced by the synovial membrane, which lines the joint capsule. It helps to reduce friction and wear between the bones that make up the joint and also provides nutrients to the cartilage that covers the bones.

When weight training is performed, the joints are placed under stress, which stimulates the synovial membrane to produce more synovial fluid. This increased production of synovial fluid helps to lubricate the joint, making it move more smoothly and easily.

Additionally, weight training can also increase the production of hyaluronan, a component of synovial fluid that helps increase the viscoelasticity of the fluid. This means the cartilage is able to resist deformation under load and recover its shape after the load is removed. This leads to improved joint flexibility and mobility.

Conversely, a sedentary lifestyle can be detrimental to the volume of synovial fluid produced. Lack of physical activity reduces the mechanical stimulation on the joints, resulting in decreased synovial fluid production. Over time, this can contribute to joint stiffness, reduced flexibility, and an increased susceptibility to joint-related problems, including osteoarthritis.

As pointed out in previous sections, synovial fluid is vital for joint health and function, providing lubrication, shock absorption, and nourishment to the joints. As we age, the production of synovial fluid diminishes, but resistance training can help stimulate its production and maintain joint health.

DON'T STOP LIFTING WEIGHTS

It's important to note that weight training should be performed properly, gradually, and progressively, starting with lower loads and gradually increasing the intensity over time. This will allow the joints to adapt to the stress and avoid injury. Also, proper form and technique is crucial to avoid joint damage. Hiring a qualified trainer is recommended but is also very difficult to find, as most trainers do not have the proper background or experience in kinesiology to facilitate proper biomechanical onboarding to clients. Choose wisely. This is part of the cost of acting upon a legitimate strength training program. If you happen to find the right one, it will be invaluable to your quality of life.

GLUCONEOGENESIS: ACCELERATING MUSCLE LOSS

Muscle Loss from Excessive Cardiovascular Training and Inadequate Nutrition

As touched on in an earlier chapter, gluconeogenesis is a metabolic process where the body converts non-carbohydrate sources, such as amino acids (derived from muscle proteins), into glucose to meet energy demands. When your dietary intake of carbohydrates and whole proteins is insufficient, gluconeogenesis can occur to maintain blood glucose levels. However, when excessive cardiovascular training is combined with inadequate nutrition, the body resorts to breaking down muscle tissue to fuel energy needs. This is radically important to understand for maintaining (and increasing) your muscle mass.

During gluconeogenesis, the body identifies amino acids obtained from muscle proteins as potential glucose sources. In the absence of sufficient carbohydrates, these amino acids undergo a series of biochemical reactions, ultimately producing glucose for essential bodily functions. While this process helps maintain blood glucose levels, it comes at the cost of breaking down muscle tissue, leading to muscle loss. The very thing you do not want.

Excessive cardiovascular training, particularly in the absence of proper nutrition, exacerbates this muscle loss phenomenon. Cardiovascular exercises, like long-distance running or intensive cycling, demand significant energy expenditure. If the body's glycogen stores are depleted due to inadequate carbohydrate intake, it seeks alternative sources to maintain energy levels, which may include breaking down muscle proteins via gluconeogenesis.

To prevent muscle loss during intense cardiovascular training, it is crucial to ensure an adequate intake of carbohydrates and whole proteins. Carbohydrates replenish glycogen stores in muscles, providing readily available energy during exercise. Consuming complex carbohydrates, such as whole grains, fruits, and vegetables, helps sustain energy levels and spares muscle tissue from being converted to glucose.

Whole proteins are equally important, as they contain all essential amino acids required for muscle repair and growth. Adequate protein intake helps preserve muscle mass, even during demanding cardiovascular workouts. Foods like lean meats, fish, legumes, and dairy are excellent sources of whole proteins that contribute to maintaining muscle integrity.

MITOCHONDRIA

The Power Supply of ATP

Mitochondria are intricate organelles within cells that serve a critical role in maintaining various cellular functions, including energy production, cell growth, and maintenance of genomic stability. One of the most pivotal functions of mitochondria is their involvement in generating adenosine triphosphate (ATP), the primary source of energy used by cells to power various physiological processes. One particularly vital part of mitochondria is the link to muscle growth in the specific role it plays in ATP storage for explosive muscle motor unit firing, as well as their role as the home of stem cells, and how the depletion of stem cells within mitochondria contributes to the aging process and eventual frailty.

Mitochondria play a crucial role in the process of cellular respiration, where glucose and oxygen are converted into ATP through a series of biochemical reactions. This energy production occurs in the inner mitochondrial membrane, specifically within the electron transport chain and oxidative phosphorylation. ATP molecules are synthesized as a result of the movement of protons across the mitochondrial inner membrane, driven by the electron transport chain. This process provides the cell with the energy needed for various activities, such as muscle contractions, nerve impulses, and metabolic processes.

Sprinters use ATP-PC as the prime energy source for 5 to 12 seconds of explosive propulsion. This is where muscle gets made in a process called hypertrophy. This is why our system of resistance training inside The FITNESS QUADRANT focuses primarily on a 6- to 15-rep range during our training.

Explosive muscle motor unit firing, which is essential for activities requiring sudden bursts of energy, heavily relies on the rapid availability of ATP. Mitochondria contribute to this process by ensuring a continuous supply of ATP in muscle cells. During high-intensity activities, such as sprinting or weightlifting, the demand for ATP increases significantly. Mitochondria respond to this demand by ramping up ATP production through oxidative phosphorylation. Consequently, well-functioning mitochondria enable muscles to contract forcefully and efficiently, supporting explosive motor unit firing essential for these activities.

Moreover, recent research has unveiled another fascinating aspect of mitochondria—their role as the home of stem cells. Stem cells are undifferentiated cells that possess the unique ability to develop into various cell types. In recent years, scientists have discovered that a small population of stem cells resides within the mitochondria. These mitochondrial-associated stem cells (MSCs) are believed to contribute to tissue repair, regeneration, and overall health. MiSCs play a role in maintaining tissue integrity and homeostasis by replenishing damaged or aging cells.

As the aging process unfolds, there is a noticeable decline in mitochondrial function and the depletion of MiSCs. This depletion of MiSCs is closely linked to the development of frailty, a condition characterized by reduced physical strength, diminished mobility, and increased susceptibility to illness. Frailty is a significant risk factor for morbidity and mortality among the elderly population. The reduction of MiSCs hampers the body's ability to regenerate and repair tissues, contributing to the decline in overall health observed in older individuals.

BROWN FAT

99% of the public has never heard of it.

Brown adipose tissue (BAT), also known as brown fat, is a specialized type of fat tissue that is primarily found in clusters along the spine and plays a crucial role in fat metabolism and thermogenesis (heat production). Several scientific studies conducted by exercise kinesiology researchers have shed light on the relationship between brown fat, physical activity, and weight management.

One study published in the *Journal of Applied Physiology* in 2021 by Dr. Michael Khoo and his team at the University of Southern California examined the effects of regular exercise on brown fat activity. The researchers found that individuals who engaged in moderate to vigorous aerobic exercise for at least 150 minutes per week had significantly higher levels of brown fat activity compared to sedentary individuals. This increased activity was associated with enhanced fat oxidation and improved metabolic health.

Another study conducted by Dr. Wouter van Marken Lichtenbelt and colleagues at Maastricht University Medical Center in the Netherlands, published in the *Journal of Clinical Investigation* in 2019, investigated the role of brown fat in cold-induced thermogenesis and its potential implications for weight management. The researchers discovered that exposure to mild cold temperatures (around 16–19°C) stimulated the activity of brown fat, leading to an increased energy expenditure and higher rates of fat oxidation.

Both studies highlight the importance of brown fat in fat metabolism and its potential role in weight management strategies. Brown fat is primarily stimulated through two mechanisms: exposure to cold temperatures and physical activity.

Cold exposure triggers the activation of brown fat through a process called non-shivering thermogenesis. When the body is exposed to cold temperatures, brown fat cells release heat to maintain core body temperature. This heat production requires the burning of energy, primarily in the form of fatty acids from stored fat tissues, leading to increased fat metabolism.

Physical activity, particularly aerobic exercise, also plays a crucial role in stimulating brown fat activity. During exercise, the body releases hormones like irisin and lactate, which have been shown to activate brown fat cells and enhance their metabolic activity. Regular exercise not only increases brown fat activity but also promotes the development of new brown fat cells, a process known as browning.

By engaging in regular aerobic exercise and incorporating mild cold exposure into daily routines, individuals can potentially stimulate their brown fat activity, leading to increased fat metabolism and improved weight management. However, it's important to note that individual responses to these interventions may vary, and a combination of a balanced diet and regular physical activity is essential for achieving and maintaining a healthy weight.

ADAPTIVE REMODELING

Increasing Joint Strength and Mobility

Joints increase in strength during weight training through a process called adaptive remodeling. This process involves the gradual strengthening of the bones, ligaments, and tendons that make up the joint.

Weight training places stress on the joints, which triggers the body to respond by laying down new bone tissue in the areas that are under stress. This results in thicker and stronger bones.

The tendons and ligaments that attach the muscles to the bones also become stronger as a result of weight training. This is because the muscles generate tension, which is transmitted through the tendons and ligaments to the bones. The tendons and ligaments adapt to this tension by becoming thicker and stronger as well.

Additionally, weight training helps to improve the stability of joints by strengthening the muscles that surround them. Stronger muscles provide better support and help to keep the joint in proper alignment, which can reduce the risk of injury.

Overall, weight training can help to increase the strength and stability of joints through adaptive remodeling, which results in stronger bones, tendons, and ligaments, and improved muscle support.

SYNCHRONOUS VERSUS ASYNCHRONOUS

How Muscle Produces Different Levels of Force

In muscle physiology, synchronous and asynchronous firing refer to the coordination and timing of muscle fiber contractions during muscle activation. These firing patterns play a crucial role in muscle hypertrophy and are particularly significant for the aging population seeking to maintain or increase muscle mass.

1. **Synchronous Firing:** Synchronous firing occurs when a group of muscle fibers within a muscle contract simultaneously, generating a powerful and coordinated force. This synchronized contraction is essential for lifting heavy weights and performing intense exercises. During synchronous firing, motor units, which are nerve-muscle fiber units, receive signals from the nervous system simultaneously, causing the muscle fibers they innervate to contract in unison. This coordinated contraction enables efficient force production and allows for lifting heavier loads during strength training exercises.

   Example: When lifting a heavy barbell during a bench press, multiple motor units in the pectoral muscles contract synchronously to generate maximum force required to lift the weight.

2. **Asynchronous Firing:** In contrast, asynchronous firing involves motor units contracting in a staggered or alternating manner. This firing pattern is more sustainable for endurance-type activities or activities that require a more sustained muscle contraction without fatigue. Asynchronous firing helps in maintaining muscle function during prolonged or repetitive movements and is crucial for activities like long-distance running or maintaining posture.

   Example: During a sustained plank exercise, different motor units in the core muscles fire asynchronously to maintain the position and support the body weight.

Importance for Hypertrophy and Aging Population:

Hypertrophy: Synchronous firing is particularly important for muscle hypertrophy, which refers to the increase in muscle size. When muscle fibers contract synchronously under substantial resistance (e.g., weightlifting with appropriate resistance), it leads to microtears in muscle fibers. The body then repairs these tears during the recovery process, resulting in muscle growth and increased muscle mass. Using adequate resistance ensures that synchronous firing occurs optimally, promoting hypertrophy.

Aging and Muscle Loss: As individuals age, there is a natural decline in muscle mass and strength known as sarcopenia. This loss of muscle mass can lead to decreased mobility, frailty, and an increased risk of falls and fractures in the elderly. Incorporating resistance training with an emphasis on synchronous firing is crucial for aging individuals. It helps counteract muscle loss by stimulating muscle fibers to contract synchronously against resistance, promoting muscle growth, strength, and overall functional ability.

Optimizing Synchronous Firing in Resistance Training: Using enough resistance during resistance training sessions *is pivotal* to trigger greater synchronous firing in muscle fibers. This, in turn, maximizes muscle activation and promotes hypertrophy. The aging population should be guided to use appropriate resistance levels in their exercises to ensure optimal synchronous firing and gain the benefits of increased muscle mass and strength.

Synchronous firing, where muscle fibers contract together, is vital for generating significant force during exercises, promoting muscle hypertrophy. For the aging population combating muscle loss, optimizing synchronous firing through resistance training is a crucial strategy to maintain or increase muscle mass, enhance strength, and improve overall quality of life

An example of *asynchronous* movements could be as small a movement like typing on a keyboard. As you type, each finger is moving independently of the others, resulting in an asynchronous muscle contraction. Or playing a guitar. As you strum or pluck the strings, your fingers are moving independently, resulting in an asynchronous muscle contraction.

Here are five more examples of asynchronous movements involving larger muscle groups:

1. Jogging / Distance Running

When jogging, muscles don't all fire at once; they fire asynchronously in a coordinated rhythm.

- Quadriceps extend the knee as the leg pushes off.

- Hamstrings and glutes fire slightly later to pull the leg through and stabilize the hip.

- Calves (Gastrocnemius/Soleus) contract on push-off, while the opposite leg prepares to land.

- Core and lower back muscles activate in alternating patterns to maintain trunk stability.

This asynchronous firing creates an efficient gait cycle that reduces fatigue and spreads load over multiple muscles.

2. Swimming (Freestyle Stroke)

During freestyle, the arms, legs, and torso don't move in unison; they fire asynchronously in a wave-like sequence.

- Latissimus dorsi and deltoids pull the arm through the water.

- Opposite arm muscles are recovering above water, firing at a different time.

- Hip flexors and glutes alternate to kick the legs in a flutter pattern.

- Obliques and core muscles rotate the torso in an offset rhythm relative to arms and legs.

This staggered muscle firing pattern allows continuous propulsion while reducing drag.

3. Cycling

Pedaling involves constant asynchronous activation of large muscle groups around the hip and knee.

- Quadriceps fire during the downward stroke (power phase).
- Hamstrings activate later in the cycle to pull upward.
- Glutes contract at hip extension points, slightly offset from quads.
- Core muscles stabilize the pelvis asynchronously with leg drive.

The offset timing keeps the pedal stroke smooth, converts circular motion into linear force, and prevents muscles from exhausting too quickly.

4. Rowing (Erg or On-Water)

Rowing is a classic example of asynchronous firing with large and medium muscle groups:

- Quadriceps extend the knees first at the catch (drive phase).
- Glutes and hamstrings then fire to extend the hips.
- Latissimus dorsi, rhomboids, and biceps activate next, pulling the handle to the chest.
- Core muscles (rectus abdominis and obliques) engage asynchronously with the pull to stabilize the spine.
- Forearm flexors contract later to grip and control the handle, but not simultaneously with the legs or glutes.

This staggered timing distributes workload and creates continuous force instead of one explosive push.

5. Climbing Stairs

Climbing stairs recruits big movers but also medium stabilizers in asynchronous patterns:

- Quadriceps fire strongly to extend the knee on the upward push.

- Gluteus maximus and hamstrings follow to extend the hip.

- Gastrocnemius and soleus (calves) fire just before toe-off, slightly delayed.

- Hip flexors (iliopsoas and rectus femoris) lift the opposite leg asynchronously with the stance leg.

- Gluteus medius and adductors act at different moments to stabilize the pelvis laterally.

This timing prevents energy waste and ensures balance while maintaining rhythm over multiple steps.

In all of these activities and examples, the involved muscles don't all fire at once because they are not being recruited for maximum force output. Instead, motor units (groups of muscle fibers and the nerves that activate them) take turns firing. Different fibers are recruited at different times in a rotating pattern.

This staggered activation reduces fatigue, allowing the runner to sustain movement for hours instead of one or two explosive, all out, hard-as-you-can movements, which I'll describe next.

Five examples of *synchronous* movements:

Now, here are five examples of *muscle-growing* synchronous strength exercises, athletic events, and a work-related activity that triggers hypertrophy. All of these movements involve heavy resistance that leads motor units to fire synchronously to produce maximum force output, which in turn drive muscle growth, or hypertrophy.

1. Olympic Sprinting & Plyometric Lower-Body Drills

Sprinting and plyos drive synchronous, explosive firing of the largest lower-body muscles.

- Glutes, hamstrings, quadriceps, and calves contract almost simultaneously to generate maximum propulsion.
- Hip flexors and core brace in sync to stabilize the trunk during rapid ground contact.

This synchronized activation recruits and overloads fast-twitch fibers, developing raw speed, power, and muscle growth.

2. Barbell or Kettlebell Deadlift

The deadlift is a prime example of synchronous firing across the posterior chain.

- Glutes, hamstrings, spinal erectors, and traps fire together to drive the lift from the floor.
- Lats and core lock in simultaneously to protect the spine.
- Grip and forearm muscles contract at the same moment to hold the load.

Because so many large groups activate at once, the deadlift produces hypertrophy, synchronous strength, and hormonal surges.

3. Clean to Press (Olympic Lift)

A full-body lift that demands powerful synchronous firing from start to finish.

- Quads, glutes, and hamstrings drive the initial pull explosively.
- Traps, deltoids, and core engage together to rack the bar.
- Shoulders, triceps, and core fire in unison to press overhead.

The clean to press integrates the entire body firing at once, producing unmatched coordination, strength, and hypertrophy.

4. Farmer's Walk with Heavy Loads

Walking under heavy load creates full-body synchronous tension.

- Forearms, grip muscles, and traps contract continuously with the shoulders and core.
- Quadriceps, hamstrings, and glutes fire together to keep each step strong and stable.

Because the entire chain contracts simultaneously underload, this move builds real-world strength, posture, and hypertrophy.

5. Heavy Sled Push / Pull Sprint

The sled push unites the lower body and core in synchronous contraction.

- Quadriceps, glutes, hamstrings, and calves fire together to drive the sled forward.
- Core and upper back lock in at the same time to maintain posture under resistance.

This simultaneous activation mimics raw labor-style power, building hypertrophy, endurance, and explosive strength.

These heavy exercises and movements are highly effective for developing synchronous strength, functional power, and muscle growth.

THE MAGIC OF INTERLEUKIN 10

How Resistance Training and Cardio Training Trigger IL-10 Release

This is one of the most profound benefits of a comprehensive fitness program. Our FITNESS QUADRANT wholly embodies and triggers this phenomenon. IL-10 is an anti-inflammatory myokine crucial for regulating immune responses, mitigating inflammation, and promoting tissue repair. Resistance training and cardiovascular exercise influence its release through mechanisms tied to the activation of the immune system and the release of myokines (muscle-derived cytokines). We'll dive into myokines a bit more in the next chapters.

1. Resistance Training and IL-10

- Mechanism:

Adequate resistance during weight training causes microtears in muscle fibers and subsequent inflammation. This process recruits immune cells (e.g., macrophages) to repair the damaged tissue.

Activated macrophages produce IL-10 to regulate the inflammatory response and prevent excessive damage.

Myokines like IL-6, which are released during resistance training, play a role in upregulating IL-10 production as a compensatory anti-inflammatory mechanism.

- Effectiveness:

Intense, high-load resistance exercises that create significant mechanical stress (e.g., heavy squats or deadlifts) are particularly effective in triggering IL-10.

2. Cardiovascular Training and IL-10

- Mechanism:

Cardiovascular exercise, especially at moderate to high intensities, induces systemic inflammation via muscle contractions, oxidative stress, and metabolic by-products.

This triggers the release of myokines such as IL-6, which indirectly stimulates IL-10 production by immune cells.

Over time, aerobic training reduces chronic low-grade inflammation by enhancing the production of IL-10, which downregulates pro-inflammatory cytokines like IL-1β, IL-6, and TNF-α.

- Effectiveness:

Continuous, steady-state cardio (e.g., running or cycling) and LifeStrong's MIT training sessions are potent stimuli for IL-10 release, with MIT showing particularly strong responses due to its acute stress on the targeted muscle chains.

Benefits of IL-10 to Health, Longevity, and Inflammation

1. Anti-inflammatory Effects

- IL-10 is a key regulator that suppresses pro-inflammatory cytokines (e.g., TNF-α, IL-1β) and inhibits the activity of inflammatory immune cells.

- It prevents excessive inflammation that can lead to chronic diseases such as arthritis, cardiovascular disease, and neurodegenerative conditions.

2. Cardiovascular Health

- By reducing systemic inflammation, IL-10 protects the vascular endothelium from damage and helps prevent atherosclerosis, hypertension, and other cardiovascular diseases.

- It enhances the repair and remodeling of blood vessels after exercise-induced stress.

3. Longevity and Aging

- Chronic low-grade inflammation, often referred to as inflammaging, accelerates aging and age-related diseases.

- IL-10 reduces this inflammation, contributing to improved health span and longevity by maintaining a balanced immune response.

4. Tissue Repair and Regeneration

- IL-10 promotes tissue healing by enhancing macrophage polarization to an anti-inflammatory phenotype (M2 macrophages) and supporting cell proliferation in damaged tissues.

- This role is critical for recovery from exercise and injury.

5. Brain Health

- IL-10 can cross the blood-brain barrier and exert neuroprotective effects by reducing neuroinflammation, which is linked to conditions such as Alzheimer's disease and depression.

- Regular exercise-induced IL-10 release contributes to better cognitive function and emotional well-being.

Both resistance and cardio training stimulate the release of IL-10, a myokine with profound health benefits. It is the essence of The FITNESS QUADRANT design. Its anti-inflammatory properties help counteract chronic inflammation, support cardiovascular and brain health, promote tissue repair, and enhance longevity. Incorporating both types of exercise into a fitness routine can optimize these benefits and contribute to a healthier, more resilient body. Absolutely amazing!

STRESS HORMONES

Stress hormones, such as cortisol and adrenaline, are released in response to stress. They are designed to help the body respond to a perceived threat, also known as the fight or flight response. However, when stress hormones are elevated for prolonged periods of time, they can have harmful effects on health.

Elevated cortisol levels can lead to an increase in appetite, weight gain, and abdominal fat, which can increase the risk of heart disease and diabetes. Prolonged high cortisol levels can also suppress the immune system, making an individual more susceptible to infections.

Adrenaline, also known as epinephrine, is a hormone that increases heart rate and blood pressure, which in turn can increase the risk of heart disease. Prolonged elevation of adrenaline levels can also lead to increased anxiety and irritability.

Additionally, stress can disrupt the balance of other hormones in the body, such as thyroid hormones, which can lead to fatigue and weight gain.

When stress hormones are elevated for prolonged periods of time, they can have harmful effects on health, including an increased risk of heart disease, diabetes, and infections. They can also disrupt the balance of other hormones in the body, leading to fatigue and weight gain. It's important to find healthy ways to manage stress, such as exercise, meditation, and therapy.

GIVE STRESS HORMONES A BEAT DOWN

Our resistance training model Modified Interval Training (MIT™) and cardio protocols are a system that strategically blends resistance training with precise cardiovascular protocols to neutralize the four most dangerous stress hormones—cortisol, adrenaline, norepinephrine, and glucagon. Resistance training helps lower chronically elevated cortisol, protecting muscle mass and preventing fat storage. Structured cardiovascular intervals regulate adrenaline and norepinephrine, keeping energy steady instead of spiking into anxiety or fatigue. Proper training intensity also balances glucagon, stabilizing blood sugar and reducing metabolic stress. The result is a powerful synergy: stress hormones are brought under control, the nervous system resets, and the body is primed for strength, resilience, and longevity. Get selfish and start prioritizing yourself a mere 3 to 4 hours a week with proper fitness protocols and stop getting robbed of a quality life.

RESISTANCE TRAINING AND NEUROGENESIS: A SECOND LOOK

Resistance training has emerged as a promising intervention for promoting neurogenesis, the process of generating new neurons in the brain. This discovery has significant implications, particularly for elderly individuals exhibiting early signs of dementia or cognitive decline. Several scientific studies have explored the effects of resistance training on neurogenesis and its potential benefits for cognitive function and brain health.

One of the seminal studies in this field was conducted by researchers at the University of British Columbia and published in the *Journal of Applied Physiology* in 2017. The study involved a group of women aged 65–75 with mild cognitive impairment (MCI), a condition that often precedes dementia. The participants were assigned to either a resistance training program or a control group. After six months of twice-weekly resistance training sessions, the researchers found significant increases in brain-derived neurotrophic factor (BDNF) levels and functional connectivity in the cognitive control networks of the brain among the resistance training group compared to the control group.

BDNF is a protein that plays a crucial role in neurogenesis, promoting the survival, growth, and differentiation of new neurons. The increased BDNF levels observed in the resistance training group suggest that this form of exercise stimulates the production of this vital protein, potentially enhancing neurogenesis and cognitive function.

Another study, published in the *Journal of the American Geriatrics Society* in 2019, investigated the effects of resistance training on cognitive function and brain structure in older adults with mild cognitive impairment. The participants underwent a 26-week resistance training program, and the researchers observed improvements in memory, executive function, and processing speed compared to a control group. Additionally, magnetic resonance imaging (MRI) scans revealed increased volume in specific brain regions associated with memory and cognitive function, suggesting that resistance training may help preserve brain structure and mitigate age-related cognitive decline.

The mechanisms underlying the positive effects of resistance training on neurogenesis are not fully understood, but several hypotheses have been proposed. One theory suggests that the mechanical stress and metabolic demands of resistance training trigger the release of growth factors, such as BDNF, insulin-like growth factor-1 (IGF-1), and vascular endothelial growth factor, which promote neurogenesis and improve brain vascular health.

Another proposed mechanism involves the regulation of inflammation and oxidative stress. Resistance training has been shown to reduce systemic inflammation and oxidative stress, both of which are known to contribute to cognitive decline and neurodegeneration. By reducing these harmful processes, resistance training may create a more favorable environment for neurogenesis and neuronal survival.

Furthermore, resistance training has been associated with improvements in sleep quality, which is essential for cognitive function and may also play a role in facilitating neurogenesis.

MYOKINES: A POWERFUL FORCE FOR LONGEVITY

What Are Myokines?

Myokines are small proteins released by muscle cells during and after physical activity, particularly strength training. When muscles contract during exercise, they produce these signaling molecules, which then enter the bloodstream and travel to various parts of the body, including the brain, fat tissue, liver, and other organs. Myokines are key to the body's response to physical stress and activity, playing a role in the repair, growth, and maintenance of tissues while also impacting overall health and disease prevention.

Myokines and Strength Training:

As we discussed above in synchronous firing patterns chapter, strength training, or resistance exercise, is one of the most potent triggers for myokine release. As muscles contract against resistance, they create mechanical tension that stimulates muscle fibers, causing them to release these beneficial proteins. Among the most well-known myokines are irisin, IL-6, and BDNF, which contribute to a wide range of health benefits.

Top Three Benefits of Myokines:

Anti-Cancer Benefits:
Myokines have shown potential in reducing cancer risk and supporting cancer treatment. They help in this regard by improving immune system function, reducing inflammation, and promoting the death of unhealthy or cancerous cells. For example, IL-6 has been linked to increased anti-tumor activity, while irisin has been shown to influence fat metabolism, potentially reducing the risk of obesity-related cancers.

Improved Muscle and Bone Health:
Myokines promote muscle growth and repair, which is critical in preserving muscle mass, especially as we age. By enhancing muscle strength, these proteins help protect against sarcopenia (age-related muscle loss), while simultaneously supporting bone health. The

release of irisin has also been shown to stimulate bone formation, which can counteract age-related bone density loss.

Metabolic Health and Weight Management:
Myokines play an important role in regulating metabolism. They increase fat oxidation and improve insulin sensitivity, which can help prevent or manage conditions like type 2 diabetes. For example, irisin has been found to turn white fat into brown fat, increasing energy expenditure and fat burning, making it easier to maintain a healthy weight.

Additional Benefits:

Cognitive Function and Brain Health:
Myokines like BDNF have been shown to improve cognitive function by enhancing brain plasticity. BDNF promotes the growth of new neurons, which is crucial for memory and learning, potentially lowering the risk of neurodegenerative diseases like Alzheimer's.

Inflammation Reduction:

Exercise-induced myokines help to modulate inflammation by suppressing pro-inflammatory cytokines and stimulating anti-inflammatory responses. This reduces the risk of chronic conditions such as cardiovascular disease and metabolic syndrome.

Cardiovascular Health:
Myokines play a role in heart health by improving blood vessel function and reducing arterial stiffness. Exercise-induced myokine release also helps maintain a healthy blood pressure and cholesterol profile, contributing to long-term cardiovascular health.

Myokines are a powerful and beneficial by-product of strength training, offering far-reaching effects on health. Not only do they help improve muscle and bone health, but they also contribute to metabolic, cardiovascular, and brain health, while offering potential anti-cancer benefits. By incorporating The FITNESS QUADRANT into your weekly lifestyle—which highlights adequate strength training into your routine—you can harness the power of myokines to optimize your health and reduce your risk of chronic diseases.

SKINNY JIMMY – PART 3

Jimmy's first 5 strength training sessions were unlike anything he had ever experienced in his forty-five years of going to the gym. He was now performing different movements with proper biomechanics at different intervals and in different patterns. He could barely make it through the 45-minute workouts. And the next day, he experienced *muscle soreness* he had never felt before—deep soreness in his lats (back), legs, glutes, and core. Notice I said muscle soreness and not joint soreness? A critical point.

So Jimmy asked, "How am I so sore when I've only worked out for 45 minutes? And how am I supposed to work out six days like this?"

I replied, "People unfortunately have never learned the science behind fitness. Things like proper biomechanics allow a maximum number of muscle fibers to recruit during each rep while at the same time allowing joints and connective tissue to remain safe through the contractions—thus minimizing GTO activation. This is why you are experiencing a higher degree of soreness—which, by the way, will temper down substantially over the next few weeks. In fact, the joints will also gain strength, range of motion, and functional integrity if they are in a safe position while the muscle is pulling on them. They too will respond to the stimuli of muscle force pulling on them. This is only one example of hundreds and part of the unseen benefits of strength training done properly. This is the bigger picture of doing this correctly."

Jimmy said, "Wow, not only do I feel it and see it, I now understand it."

The next step was connecting the nutrition (N) quadrant to the resistance (R) training quadrant. I asked Jimmy, "When we went over your nutrition plan, did you understand how vital your protein intake is?"

He replied, "I think so, but I am still a little confused on this whole protein thing. Isn't protein all the same? I mean, it says there is protein in the bread that I eat. Should I be counting that as my daily protein intake?"

"That's a great question," I replied, "and one that confuses 99% of the public and the people I train. They don't realize that there is a major difference between whole protein versus incomplete protein.

"Protein comes in two basic forms. Incomplete and whole. Bread and rice are examples of foods that contain incomplete proteins. Incomplete proteins will not repair and build muscle fibers. We are after whole proteins for our intake throughout the day. A whole protein contains the nine essential amino acids the body cannot produce that count and matter when you are meeting the demand of muscle growth and maintenance. No exceptions. Whole protein is found in eggs, red meat, chicken, fish, dairy, and protein powder or quality protein supplements. This is a staple lesson of the Nutrition quadrant and a vital phase of triggering growth in your body. There needs to be an adequate amount of whole protein ingested daily through your diet to meet the metabolic demand and the tissue repair demand. If you don't get enough of it, you will continue to lose muscle.

"For you, Jimmy, your amount will be about 130 grams minimum daily to start. This will ensure you have enough to support your body in building and repairing muscle. Once you get your protein requirements right, we can move on to carbohydrate and fat intake during the next lesson."

CHAPTER 6

THE PSYCHOLOGY OF FORMING HABITS

The psychology of habit formation is a fascinating area of study that explores how habits, both good and bad, are formed and maintained. Habits are automatic behavioral patterns that are acquired through repetition and become ingrained in our daily lives. Understanding the process of habit formation can be useful for promoting positive behaviors, such as regular exercise and breaking unhealthy habits.

Research suggests that forming habits can take anywhere from a few weeks to several months, depending on various factors. One influential study conducted by Phillippa Lally and colleagues at University College London examined the time it takes for individuals to form new habits. They found that, on average, it took participants about 66 days to establish a new habit, but the time frame varied widely, ranging from 18 to 254 days. This indicates that the duration of habit formation is highly individual and can depend on factors such as motivation, consistency, and the complexity of the behavior.

The process of habit formation typically involves several stages:

1. Cue: A trigger or cue that initiates the habit loop. It can be a specific time, location, emotion, or action that prompts the behavior.

2. Routine: The actual behavior or action that constitutes the habit. This can be a simple or complex action that is consistently performed in response to the cue.

3. Reward: The positive reinforcement or benefit associated with the behavior. Rewards can be intrinsic (e.g., a sense of accomplishment) or extrinsic (e.g., a treat or praise), and they play a crucial role in reinforcing the habit loop.

By understanding these stages, individuals can intentionally shape their habits. Here are some strategies that can help in forming and maintaining healthy habits:

1. Start small: Begin with achievable and manageable goals to build momentum and establish a sense of success.

2. Consistency: Consistently repeat the desired behavior to reinforce the habit loop and make it more automatic over time.

3. Environment design: Modify your environment to make the desired behavior easier to perform and the cues more prominent. For example, placing exercise equipment in a visible area or setting out workout clothes can serve as cues for exercising.

4. Behavioral tracking: Keep track of your progress and celebrate milestones to maintain motivation and reinforce the habit loop.

5. Accountability and support: Seek social support from friends, family, or groups with similar goals to help yourself stay accountable and provide encouragement.

Remember, breaking bad habits can be challenging, but it is possible by applying similar principles in reverse. Identifying the cues and replacing the routine with a healthier behavior, while still providing a reward, can help shift you away from unwanted habits.

In the context of fitness habits, it is important to note that habit formation can be influenced by various factors, including the complexity of the behavior, individual differences, and personal circumstances. The duration required to establish a routine fitness habit can vary among individuals. Consistency and persistence are key factors in forming sustainable fitness habits, and it is recommended to focus on gradual progress rather than expecting immediate results.

Overall, understanding the psychology of habit formation can empower individuals to intentionally shape their behaviors and promote positive habits while breaking detrimental ones.

CHAPTER 7

OSTEOPOROSIS

THE FEMALE NIGHTMARE

Osteoporosis, characterized by reduced bone mineral density (BMD) and increased fracture risk, is a significant health issue among women aged 35 to 85. Studies indicate that women may lose up to 45% of their bone and muscle mass between these ages without interventions. The prevalence of osteoporosis increases sharply after menopause, with around 25% of postmenopausal women being affected by the disease.

Factors Contributing to Bone Loss

- **Age-Related Decline:** Bone loss accelerates after age 35 due to hormonal changes, particularly reduced estrogen levels post-menopause.

- **Lifestyle Factors:** Sedentary behavior, low calcium and vitamin D intake, and smoking exacerbate bone density loss.

The Role of Resistance Training for Brittle Bones

Resistance training is your best weapon against brittle bones, not more drugs. It is a proven intervention to mitigate bone density loss. Studies show that as little as two hours of high-impact resistance training weekly can increase BMD at key skeletal sites such as the spine, hips, and femur. This effect occurs because mechanical loading stimulates bone remodeling and strengthens musculoskeletal support, reducing fall and fracture risks. Notable benefits include:

- **Increased BMD:** Gains in BMD were observed in postmenopausal women engaging in structured strength training programs.

- **Functional Improvements:** Resistance training also enhances muscle strength, balance, and overall physical function, further reducing osteoporosis-related risks.

Trends in Osteoporosis

Global data shows rising osteoporosis cases due to aging populations. In the US, the incidence of osteoporosis in women over 50 increased significantly from the 1990s to 2020.

This evidence underscores the importance of preventive measures like proper resistance training, not just the typical advice from your doctor: "You need to exercise." What the hell does that mean, Doc? And yes, proper nutrition and then nutritional supplementation combat osteoporosis very effectively.

Osteoporosis Prevalence by Age Group

The prevalence of osteoporosis increases sharply with age, particularly after menopause. In the 75–85 age group, approximately 65% of women are affected.

Impact of Resistance Training on Bone Mineral Density (BMD):

Engaging in resistance training leads to measurable improvements in BMD, with gains of up to 7% observed after 12 months of consistent training.

The following charts illustrate two key aspects related to osteoporosis and bone health:

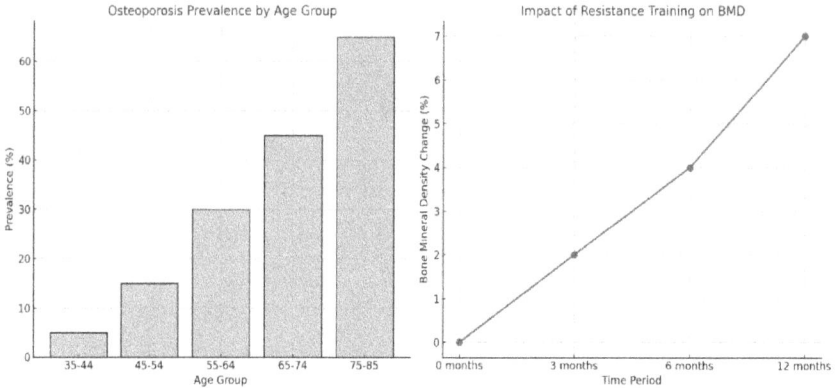

These visualizations emphasize the growing risk of osteoporosis with age and the importance of proactive measures like resistance training to enhance bone strength and reduce fracture risk.

MUSCLE MASS: A MARKER OF LONGEVITY

I have mentioned this repeatedly throughout this book. It's that important. Maintaining muscle mass is a critical marker for longevity, directly influencing metabolic health, physical function, and overall resilience against chronic diseases and age-related decline. Research highlights the profound link between muscle mass and lifespan, with resistance training being the primary and most effective way to build and preserve muscle.

The Role of Muscle Mass in Longevity

1. Metabolic Health:

   Muscle acts as a glucose sink, helping regulate blood sugar levels and reduce the risk of insulin resistance and type 2 diabetes. Research in *Diabetes Care* confirms that greater muscle mass is associated with improved metabolic function and reduced mortality risk. You cannot afford to lose muscle as you age.

2. Physical Independence:

    Muscle mass supports mobility and reduces the risk of falls and fractures, which are significant mortality factors in older adults. A study published in *The Journals of Gerontology* found that individuals with higher muscle mass experienced fewer mobility-related complications.

3. Inflammation and Immunity:

    Muscle produces myokines, anti-inflammatory molecules that combat chronic low-grade inflammation—a driver of aging and diseases like Alzheimer's, cardiovascular disease, and cancer.

4. Cardiovascular Benefits:

    Research in *Circulation* shows that higher muscle strength correlates with lower cardiovascular risk, improving overall life expectancy.

The Unique Role of Resistance Training

Resistance training is the only reliable method to add muscle mass to the human body. Unlike aerobic exercises, which primarily improve cardiovascular endurance, resistance training stimulates muscle protein synthesis and combats muscle atrophy.

How Resistance Training Works:

-   By creating microscopic tears in muscle fibers, resistance exercises (e.g., weightlifting, bodyweight movements) trigger repair and growth, leading to increased muscle size and strength.

-   Consistent training enhances neuromuscular efficiency, improves bone density, and strengthens connective tissues, all contributing to longevity.

Key Studies:

1. The Framingham Heart Study:

    Highlighted the link between muscle mass and survival rates, showing that individuals with higher muscle mass live longer regardless of fat mass

2. Harvard Health Review:

    Found that resistance training significantly improves muscle mass, reduces sarcopenia (age-related muscle loss), and extends health span in older adults

Longevity Studies: Resistance and Cardio Training

Regular resistance training—done properly—and cardiovascular exercise have been shown to have a significant positive impact on longevity and quality of life in later years. Numerous studies have highlighted the benefits of consistent physical activity, particularly in older adults. Here's a detailed summary of recent research on this topic, including relevant statistics:

1. Resistance Training and Longevity: A study published in the *British Journal of Sports Medicine* in 2021 analyzed data from over 99,000 participants aged 42–81 years. The researchers found that engaging in resistance training was associated with a 10%–20% lower risk of all-cause mortality compared to those who did not engage in strength training. Additionally, the risk of mortality decreased further with higher volumes of resistance training.

2. Cardiovascular Exercise and Longevity: A large-scale study published in the *Journal of the American Heart Association* in 2020 involved over 116,000 participants aged 40–85 years. The results showed that individuals who engaged in moderate to vigorous aerobic exercise had a 21%–23% lower risk of mortality compared to those who were inactive. The benefits

were observed across various age groups, including older adults.

3. Combined Exercise and Longevity: A systematic review and meta-analysis published in the *British Journal of Sports Medicine* in 2022 analyzed data from over thirty-six studies and nearly 2 million participants. The analysis revealed that individuals who adhered to both aerobic and resistance training recommendations had a 40% lower risk of all-cause mortality compared to those who were inactive. The risk reduction was even more significant (47%) for those who exceeded the recommended exercise levels.

4. Quality of Life: A study published in the *Journal of Aging and Physical Activity* in 2020 examined the effects of a 12-week resistance training program on quality of life in older adults aged 65–80 years. The researchers observed significant improvements in physical function, mobility, and overall quality of life scores among the participants who underwent resistance training.

5. Cognitive Function: A systematic review and meta-analysis published in the *Journal of Cognitive Enhancement* in 2021 analyzed data from twenty-eight studies involving older adults aged 60 years and above. The analysis revealed that regular aerobic exercise and resistance training were associated with improved cognitive function, including better performance in areas such as executive function, memory, and processing speed.

According to the WHO, physical inactivity is a leading risk factor for premature mortality worldwide, contributing to an estimated 33.2 million deaths annually.

A study published in *The Lancet* in 2022 estimated that regular physical activity could increase life expectancy by an average of 8.2 years globally.

The CDC reports that only around 23% of adults aged 65 and older meet the recommended levels of aerobic and muscle-strengthening physical activity.

The consistent findings from these studies and reviews underscore the importance of regular resistance training and cardiovascular exercise for promoting longevity and enhancing quality of life in older adults. The data suggests that engaging in a combination of aerobic and strength training activities can significantly reduce the risk of premature mortality and improve physical, cognitive, and overall well-being. However, it's important to note that individual responses may vary, and proper guidance from healthcare professionals is recommended when starting or modifying an exercise program, especially for older adults or those with pre-existing conditions.

Muscle mass and strength have emerged as crucial indicators of healthy aging, particularly among individuals aged 65 and above. Sarcopenia, the age-related loss of skeletal muscle mass and function, has been recognized as a significant threat to the well-being and independence of older adults. Recent medical research has shed light on the importance of maintaining muscle health and the potential benefits of resistance training in mitigating the effects of sarcopenia.

An additional key study in this field is the *Longitudinal Aging Study Amsterdam (LASA)*, which has been ongoing since 1992. This study has provided valuable insights into the relationship between muscle mass, strength, and various health outcomes in older adults. The findings suggest that low muscle mass and strength are associated with an increased risk of functional limitations, falls, fractures, and even mortality (Visser et al., 2005).

Another notable study, published in *JAMA* in 2018, investigated the association between grip strength and cardiovascular disease and mortality risk in older adults (Leong et al., 2018). The researchers found that lower grip strength was independently associated with an increased risk of cardiovascular events and mortality, highlighting the importance of maintaining muscle strength in aging populations.

Sarcopenia, as mentioned in the first part of this book, is the age-related loss of skeletal muscle mass and function, and has been recognized as a significant threat to the well-being and independence of older adults. A systematic review and meta-analysis published in the *Journal of Cachexia, Sarcopenia and Muscle* in 2019 (Shafiee et al., 2019) estimated the global prevalence of sarcopenia to be around 10% in individuals aged 60 years and older, with higher rates among those aged 80 and above.

The consequences of sarcopenia can be severe, including an increased risk of falls, functional impairment, disability, and even mortality. A study published in the *Journal of the American Geriatrics Society* (Cawthon et al., 2015) found that sarcopenia was associated with a higher risk of hospitalization and increased healthcare costs, underscoring the economic burden of this condition.

Fortunately, resistance training has emerged as a promising intervention for combating sarcopenia and promoting muscle health in older adults. A systematic review and meta-analysis published in the *British Journal of Sports Medicine* (Fragala et al., 2019) examined the effects of resistance training on muscle mass, strength, and physical function in older adults. The results demonstrated significant improvements in all three outcomes, with greater benefits observed in individuals with lower baseline muscle mass or strength.

Furthermore, a study published in *JAMA* in 2019 (Borde et al., 2019) investigated the effects of a progressive resistance training program on muscle strength and physical function in older adults with mild to moderate frailty. The findings showed significant improvements in muscle strength, gait speed, and physical function, suggesting that resistance training can help mitigate the effects of frailty and promote functional independence in aging populations.

Recent medical research has highlighted the importance of muscle mass and strength as markers of healthy aging in individuals aged 65 and older. Sarcopenia poses a significant threat to the well-being and independence of older adults, increasing the risk of functional limitations, falls, fractures, and mortality.

However, resistance training has emerged as a vital solution to combat muscle loss and promote muscle health, offering substantial benefits in terms of muscle mass, strength, and physical function.

As the global population continues to age, addressing sarcopenia and promoting muscle health through resistance training should be a priority in maintaining the quality of life and independence of older adults.

SKINNY JIMMY – PART 4
THE REBUILT JIMMY

This is a demonstration of how The FITNESS QUADRANT changes lives. Jimmy stuck to it vigorously for years.

At age 68, he had gained 20 pounds of muscle—a.k.a. lean body weight—in his first sixteen months. He now weighs approximately 171 pounds and still has under 10% body fat. Remember, he started at 149 pounds!

Jimmy is now 71 years old. He is in the best shape of his life. He's much stronger, approximately 20 pounds heavier (mostly muscle), and now has zero knee, lower back, or shoulder issues. His lower body—glutes and thighs—are visibly much bigger. No more toothpick legs! His core is like steel—balanced and stronger than ever in every plane, 360 degrees of strength, because of our consistent core training that involves every plane. People are in disbelief when they see him train in the gym. They can't believe he is 71. He out-trains most 45-year-olds and is also stronger than most.

But the impact from The FITNESS QUADRANT ecosystem is life changing for him. His new wellness lifestyle we have designed for him (and everyone else that onboards with us) has allowed him to walk the 500+ miles of the famed Camino in Europe multiple times with ease and also has ushered in his morning swims at the ocean or lake that are miles long. What a way to enjoy your 70s! He is the epitome of The FITNESS QUADRANT. And he's not the only one in our network of clients.

It's been many years since Jimmy started training with me at this point. Full-blown system, three days per week high-level resistance training sessions, with one to two day per week cardio (he didn't need to lose any more fat!). We've scaled up his nutrition and moved his metabolic set point a few times, so his caloric intake is now much higher than when we started. Same food types (always), but just a lot more of them. His starting calorie allotment was approximately 1,900 per day, and he could barely eat that much in the beginning. We are now at about 2,100 calories per day: 40% protein, 30% carbohydrates, and 30% fats.

One of the greatest things that Jimmy has acquired is knowledge. He can walk into any gym anywhere in the world (including cruise ships!) and continue his health journey. In fact, he just got back from a fourteen-day trip that was on a ship and covered Italy, Greece, and Türkiye. The ship had very little gym equipment. His words to me were, "It didn't matter. I was able to do full-blown workouts anyway." That is what I'm talking about! Jimmy could work out on a mountainside and still train like a pro. He is now certainly in the top 2%–3% of the of the competency pyramid. And that's true for pretty much all of my clients who stick with the program. The FITNESS QUADRANT and MIT training method is a game changer.

CHAPTER 8

IMAGINE IF WE COULD MAKE THIS HAPPEN…

…a transformative public health initiative where overweight and sedentary individuals in the US commit to a basic proper fitness and nutrition program.

I researched statistics and built a hypothetical scenario.

This was based on the national cost savings and health benefits in the form of life extension if people that are considered obese and sedentary were to start a proper basic fitness and nutrition regimen. Based off The FITNESS QUADRANT system, I created a hypothetical overweight person who lost 20 to 25 pounds of excess fat, gained 3 pounds of muscle, got off 90% of their prescription drugs, and began to eat ultra healthy, unprocessed foods with very low sugar and adequate whole proteins.

HYPOTHETICAL SCENARIO: NATIONAL COST SAVINGS AND HEALTH BENEFITS

Projected Health Benefits

1. **Life Extension**
   o **Weight Loss and Fitness:** Losing 20–25 pounds of excess fat significantly lowers the risk of cardiovascular diseases, type 2 diabetes, and metabolic syndrome. Studies suggest

that reducing obesity-related risks can extend life expectancy by three to ten years for previously obese individuals.

o **Improved Diet:** Transitioning to whole, nutrient-dense foods containing minimal sugar reduces chronic inflammation, enhances immune function, and protects against diseases such as cancer, Alzheimer's, and liver disease.

2. Reduced Chronic Disease Burden

o **Type 2 Diabetes:** With weight loss and improved insulin sensitivity, an estimated 80% of type 2 diabetes cases could be reversed or put into remission.

o **Cardiovascular Health:** Lowered blood pressure, improved cholesterol levels, and reduced arterial plaque formation drastically reduce the incidence of heart attacks and strokes.

o **Joint Health:** Decreasing weight alleviates pressure on joints, reducing arthritis symptoms and the need for joint replacement surgeries.

Economic Savings

1. Reduced Healthcare Costs

o **Prescription Drug Reduction:** Obese individuals often require medications for hypertension, diabetes, and cholesterol management. Reducing drug use by 90% could save approximately $6,000 per person annually (based on CDC estimates of average medication costs). With 42% of the adult US population classified as obese (~100 million people), this could lead to $600 billion in annual savings on prescription drugs alone.

2. Fewer Hospital Visits:
Healthier individuals are far less likely to need costly surgeries, hospitalization, or emergency care. For example, the average cost of a diabetes-related hospitalization is $17,000.

3. Increased Productivity

o Healthier individuals take fewer sick days, have higher energy levels, and show increased workplace productivity. This could add an estimated $150 billion annually to the economy due to improved workforce performance (based on CDC productivity loss estimates related to obesity).

4. Reduced Disability Claims

o By preventing or reversing chronic conditions, long-term disability claims related to obesity and its complications (e.g., mobility issues, diabetes-related amputations) could decrease by up to 75%, further reducing national healthcare and insurance costs.

Population-Wide Health Impact

1. Chronic Disease Reduction:

o 80% reduction in type 2 diabetes cases.

o 50% decrease in heart disease and stroke rates.

o 40% lower cancer rates due to improved diet and reduced inflammation.

2. Weight-Related Mortality Decline:

o Approximately 300,000 deaths annually in the US are attributed to obesity. If obesity rates dropped significantly, this number could fall by more than 70%, saving 200,000 lives annually.

3. Enhanced Quality of Life:

o Improved mental health due to exercise and better nutrition.

o Increased physical mobility and independence for millions of older adults.

This hypothetical national shift could save over $750 billion annually in healthcare costs and lost productivity, while extending the average life expectancy of millions by five to ten years. The ripple effects— fewer chronic diseases, healthier communities, and a more robust economy—would make this initiative one of the most impactful public health interventions in modern history, and it would make people healthier and happier.

CLOSING THOUGHTS

Fitness never stops. It never sleeps. It's either improving or imploding. If you capture the essence of *The GOAT Within*, this book will never end for you. There is no ending. This is forever material. The final never-ending chapter is you in action.

The process of supercharging your health is easy when you know how to do it correctly. The process is very difficult—nearly impossible—if you don't. Remember, we talked about paying a price at the beginning of this book. The price is far greater if you avoid an adequate, complete fitness and wellness system in your story line. It's your story and you control it.

As we covered in the first section, step one is eliminating toxic foods and products from your life (and your family's life) if you want to thrive. The toxic system of chemical foods and products is not going to change. *You are the only one who can change it*. There is way too much dirty money to be made—billions upon billions—by big businesses that prioritize profits over people, and then they secure their spots by getting connected with politicians who write the laws, and in return, need the greenbacks to win elections and stay in power. It's a cycle that will never be broken. It's too powerful.

So when your personal light bulb gets turned on—that personal power button within you—you'll decide to make the necessary changes to live in a growth mode. You'll stop accepting what has become a normal habit—engaging in blind behavior that just results in a losing battle when it comes to your health, quality of life, and longevity. You'll then start the process of breaking free from the herd. This is step one. Get hungry. Turn on the light. Punch your personal strength and wellness ticket every week, rain or shine.

Next, you add in step two—The FITNESS QUADRANT—the triggers of metabolic growth through resistance training, earth-based nutrition, and cardio work that you stay consistent at. Then, the science takes hold, and you begin to flourish into a strong, energetic, durable human being. A Viking. A stallion. A female warrior. A strong powerful leader that people want to emulate. Be that example. Find the GOAT within you. It's there, waiting for you to open the door.

The GOAT formula will make you unstoppable:

- **Avoid toxic foods and products:** These destroy your vital systems
- **Resistance train:** Your muscle stimulus to gain and maintain muscle
- **Nutrition choices:** Make earth food and whole proteins a priority
- **Cardiovascular work:** A strong circulatory system is gold (heart and lungs)
- **Recovery:** Learn how to recharge your battery and repair tissue
- **Get a posse:** True fitness friends to build positive vibes and mental connectivity

A huge thanks to all of you. I'll see you in the gym! And remember…

God gifted you your divine body. Treat it with the highest respect and highest honor, for he is the king of kings. And as we always say in our church—God is good all the time, and all the time, God is good.

Stay connected with us and find more information, tips, and programs at:

www.fitnessquadrant.net

www.skool.com/lifestrong/about

LINKEDIN: linkedin.com/in/coach-timothy-ward

INSTAGRAM: FITNESSQUADRANT

ABOUT THE AUTHOR

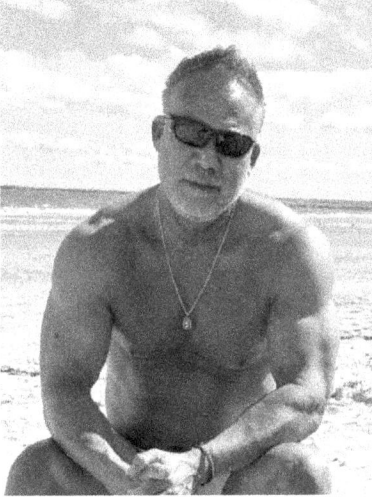

Timothy Ward is an expert fitness and longevity trainer, Author, health and motivational coach/speaker with over 30 years of expertise in exercise and nutrition sciences.

As a Master Trainer, Timothy has designed thousands of transformative fitness programs, earning a reputation as a pioneer in the industry.

He is the creator of the Fitness Quadrant™, a revolutionary framework for sustainable health and longevity, and the innovative Modified Interval Training (MIT) Method, which has redefined workout efficiency with comprehensive workouts done in 45 minutes that results in more muscle gain, fat loss, and peak performance. His system *is* the proven strategy for many men and women 40 and older to strengthen the three critical longevity markers—muscle mass, heart strength, and metabolic health.

With decades of experience, Timothy has empowered countless individuals to unlock their full physical potential and get to their personal GOAT WITHIN.

He is joined in his lifelong personal fitness journey by his wife and workout partner Julie, and his two sons Maxwell and Jesse, who also are bright examples of ultra fit young men in their 20s.

CONNECT AND LEARN WITH US:

www.fitnessquadrant.net

www.skool.com/lifestrong/about

LINKEDIN: linkedin.com/in/coach-timothy-ward

INSTAGRAM: FITNESSQUADRANT

ACKNOWLEDGMENTS

To the people who made me, saved me, pushed me, encouraged me, inspired me, and yelled at me occasionally, I cannot possibly thank you enough. So many in my life have made me a better person. I'll start with my wife, Julie, who is a rock-solid loving partner, person, and incredible mom to my two gifts from God—Maxwell, who is way smarter than me, and Jesse, who is *way* calmer and more insightful than me. I love you guys.

And to my unbelievable long-time clients—what a ride it's been. Sorry if I forgot some of you:

> Joe, Jay, Anthony, John, Bill, Sharry, Mark, Tarek, Wayne, Jeff, Nick, Margie, Amelia, Mike, David, Jay, Drew, Ken (Alfred), Tom, Kevin, David, Andrew, Bruce, Betsy, John S., Julie, Michelle, Daniela, Jill, Jerry, Patrick, Ben, Cody, Hunter, Joey, Dan F, Scott R, Mark, Bethany, Caleb, Chase boys, Quinn and Jesse, Howie—I miss you—and to my rooted group, Tonia and George, Bruce and Cindy, David and Beth, Jim and Tara, and then my longtime friends, Ronnie and Big Chad. Much love to all you guys.

Thanks to the workout crews—all of you—for sticking it out and trusting me for years on end. Your growth and fitness success has been nothing short of amazing. And you have held me together on those tough early winter mornings more than you realize! God bless you.

And most of all, I thank God for the gifts he has bestowed upon me and the courage he has put inside of me. Thanks for shining your light on me in my darkest moments. I have immense never-ending gratitude to You.